LECTURE NOTES ON
MEDICAL ENTOMOLOGY

To Thursday

Lecture Notes on
Medical Entomology

M. W. SERVICE
BSc PhD DSc FI Biol.
Reader in Medical Entomology
Liverpool School of Tropical Medicine
Liverpool, England

BLACKWELL SCIENTIFIC PUBLICATIONS
OXFORD LONDON EDINBURGH
BOSTON PALO ALTO MELBOURNE

© 1986 by
Blackwell Scientific Publications
Editorial offices:
Osney Mead, Oxford, OX2 0EL
8 John Street, London, WC1N 2ES
23 Ainslie Place, Edinburgh, EH3 6AJ
52 Beacon Street, Boston
  Massachusetts 02108, USA
667 Lytton Avenue, Palo Alto
  California 94301, USA
107 Barry Street, Carlton
  Victoria 3053, Australia

First published 1986

Printed and bound in Great Britain
by Butler & Tanner Ltd,
Frome and London

DISTRIBUTORS

USA
  Blackwell Mosby Book Distributors
  11830 Westline Industrial Drive
  St Louis, Missouri 63141

Canada
  The C.V. Mosby Company
  5240 Finch Avenue East,
  Scarborough, Ontario

Australia
  Blackwell Scientific Publications
    (Australia) Pty Ltd
  107 Barry Street
  Carlton, Victoria 3053

British Library
Cataloguing in Publication Data

Service, M.W.
  Lecture notes on medical
    entomology.
  1. Arthropod vectors
  I. Title
  595'.2   RA641.A7

ISBN 0-632-01525-X

Contents

Acknowledgement

Fig. 1.13 was drawn by M. G. Yates, and was originally used by Edward Arnold, London, in their *Studies in Biology* series, no. 167.

Chapter 1
Introduction to the Mosquitoes

There are some 3200 species of mosquitoes belonging to 37 genera, all contained in the family Culicidae. This family is divided into three subfamilies: Toxorhynchitinae, Anophelinae (anophelines) and Culicinae (culicines). Mosquitoes have a world-wide distribution; they occur throughout the tropical and temperate regions and extend their range northwards into the arctic circle, the only area from which they are absent is Antarctica. They are found at elevations of 5500 m and in mines at depths of 1250 m below sea level.

The most important man-biting mosquitoes belong to the genera *Anopheles*, *Culex*, *Aedes*, *Mansonia*, *Haemagogus* and *Sabethes*.

Anopheles species, as well as transmitting malaria are also vectors of filariasis (*Wuchereria bancrofti*, *Brugia malayi* and *B. timori*) and a few arboviruses. Certain *Culex* species transmit *Wuchereria bancrofti* and a variety of arboviruses. The genus *Aedes* contains important vectors of yellow fever, dengue, encephalitis viruses and many other arboviruses, and also vectors of *Wuchereria bancrofti* and *Brugia malayi*, while *Mansonia* species transmit *Brugia malayi* and sometimes *Wuchereria bancrofti* and a few arboviruses. *Haemagogus* and *Sabethes* mosquitoes are vectors of yellow fever and a few other arboviruses in South and Central America.

Several mosquitoes in other genera have also been incriminated as vectors of various arboviruses. Moreover, many species, although not carriers of any disease, can nevertheless be troublesome because of the serious biting nuisances they cause.

EXTERNAL MORPHOLOGY OF MOSQUITOES

Mosquitoes possess only one pair of functional wings, the fore wings. The hind wings are represented by a pair of small, knob-like halteres. Mosquitoes are distinguished from other flies of a

1

somewhat similar shape and size by: (i) the possession of a conspicuous forward projecting proboscis; (ii) the presence of numerous appressed scales on the thorax, legs, abdomen and wing veins; and (iii) a fringe of scales along the posterior margin of the wings.

Mosquitoes are slender and relatively small insects, usually measuring about 4-6 mm in length. Some species, however, can be as small as 2-3 mm while others may be as long as 10 mm. The body is distinctly divided into a head, thorax and abdomen.

The head has a conspicuous pair of kidney-shaped compound eyes. Between the eyes arises a pair of filamentous and segmented antennae. In females the antennae have whorls of short hairs (that is pilose antennae), but in males, with a few exceptions in genera of no medical importance, the antennae have many long hairs giving them a feathery or plumose appearance. Mosquitoes can thus be conveniently sexed by examination of the antennae: individuals with feathery antennae are males, while those with only short and rather inconspicuous antennal hairs are females (see Fig. 1.13). Just below the antennae are a pair of palps which may be long or short and dilated or pointed at their tips, depending on the sex of the adults and whether adults are anophelines or culicines (see Fig. 1.13). Arising between the palps is the single elongated proboscis, which contains the piercing mouth parts of the mosquito. In mosquitoes the proboscis characteristically projects forwards (Fig. 1.1).

The thorax is covered, dorsally and laterally, with scales which may be dull or shiny, white, brown, black or almost any colour. It is the arrangement of black and white, or coloured, scales on the dorsal surface of the thorax that gives many species (especially those of the genus *Aedes*) distinctive patterns (see Fig. 3.3).

The wings are long and relatively narrow and the number and arrangement of the wing veins is virtually the same for all mosquito species (see Fig.1.1). The veins are covered with scales which are usually brown, black, white or creamy yellow, but more brightly coloured scales may occasionally be present. The shape of the scales and the pattern they form differs considerably both between genera and species of mosquitoes. Scales also project as a fringe along the posterior border of the wings. In life the wings of resting mosquitoes are placed across each other over the abdomen in the fashion of a closed pair of scissors. The legs of the mosquito are long and slender and are covered with scales which

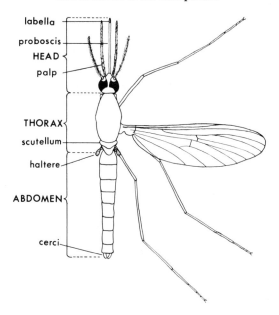

Fig. 1.1 Diagrammatic representation of a female anopheline mosquito.

are usually brown, black or white and may be arranged in patterns, often in the form of rings (see Fig. 3.4). The tarsus terminates in, usually, a pair of toothed or simple claws. Some genera such as *Culex* have a pair of small fleshy pulvilli (Fig. 1.2) at the end of the tarsus.

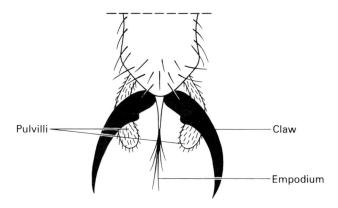

Fig. 1.2 Last segment of the tarsus of a *Culex* mosquito showing claws, hairlike empodium and fleshy pulvilli.

In mosquitoes of the subfamily Culicinae, the segmented abdomen is usually covered dorsally and ventrally with mostly brown, blackish or whitish scales. In the Anophelinae, however, the abdomen is almost, or entirely, devoid of these scales. The last abdominal segment of the female mosquitoe terminates in a small pair of finger-like cerci, whereas in the males a pair of prominent claspers, comprising part of the male genitalia, are present.

In unfed mosquitoes the abdomen is thin and slender but after females have bitten a suitable host and taken a blood-meal (only females bite), the abdomen becomes greatly distended and resembles a red oval balloon. When the abdomen is full of developing eggs it is also dilated, but is whitish and not red in appearance.

Mouthparts and salivary glands

The mouthparts are collectively known as the proboscis. In mosquitoes the proboscis is elongate and projects conspicuously forwards in both sexes—although males do not bite. The largest component of the mouthparts is the long and flexible gutter-shaped labium which terminates in a pair of small flap-like structures called the labella. In cross-section the labium is seen to almost enrircle all the other components of the mouthparts (Fig. 1.3) and serves as a protective sheath. The individual components are held close together in life and only become partially separated during blood-feeding, or when they are teased apart for examination as illustrated in Fig. 1.4.

The uppermost structure, the labrum, is slender, pointed and grooved along its ventral surface. In between this 'upper roof'

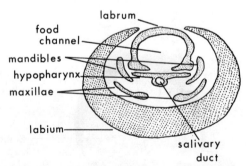

Fig. 1.3 Diagram of a transverse section through the proboscis of a mosquito showing the components of the mouthparts and the food channel.

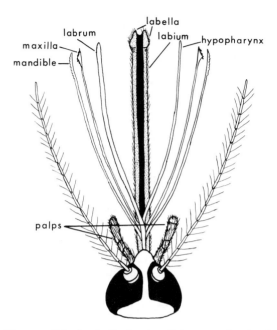

Fig. 1.4 Diagram of the head of a female culicine mosquito showing the components of the mouthparts dissected from the labium.

(labrum) and 'lower gutter' (labium) are five needle-like structures, namely, a lower pair of toothed maxillae, an upper pair of mandibles, which are more finely toothed, and finally a single untoothed, hollow stylet called the hypopharynx. When a female mosquito bites a host the labella, at the tip of the fleshy labium, are placed on the skin and the labium which cannot pierce the skin curves backwards. This allows the paired mandibles, paired maxillae, labrum and hypopharynx to penetrate the host's skin. Saliva from a pair of trilobed salivary glands, situated ventrally in the anterior part of the thorax, is pumped down the hypopharynx. Saliva contains anticoagulins and/or haemagglutinins which prevent the blood from clotting and obstructing the mouthparts as it is sucked up into the space formed by the apposition of the labrum and the other piercing mouthparts.

Although male mosquitoes have a proboscis, the mandibles and maxillae are reduced in size or are absent and so males cannot bite.

LIFE-CYCLE

Blood-feeding and the gonotrophic cycle

Most mosquitoes mate shortly after emergence from the pupa. Sperm, passed by the male into the spermotheca of the female, usually serve to fertilise all eggs laid during her lifetime, thus only one mating and insemination per female is required. With a few exceptions, a female mosquito must bite a host and take a blood-meal to obtain the necessary nutrients for the development of the eggs in the ovaries. This is the normal procedure and is referred to as anautogenous development. A few species, however, can develop the first batch of eggs without a blood-meal. This process is called autogenous development. The speed of digestion of the blood-meal depends on temperature and in most tropical species takes only 2–3 days, but in colder, temperate countries blood digestion may take as long as 7–14 days.

After a blood-meal the mosquitoe's abdomen is dilated and bright red in colour, but some hours later the abdomen becomes a much darker red. As the blood is digested and the white eggs in the ovaries enlarge, the abdomen becomes whitish posteriorly and dark reddish anteriorly. This condition represents a mid-point in blood digestion and ovarian development, and the mosquito is referred to as being half-gravid (Fig. 1.5). Eventually all blood is digested and the abdomen becomes dilated and whitish due to the formation of fully developed eggs (Fig. 1.5). The female is now said to be gravid and she searches for suitable larval

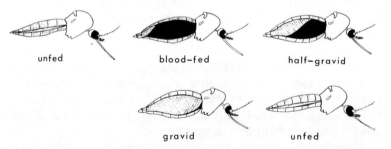

Fig. 1.5 Diagrammatic representation of the gonotrophic cycle of a female mosquito. Each cycle starts with an unfed adult, passing through a blood-fed, half-gravid and gravid condition. Then after oviposition the female is again unfed and seeks another blood-meal.

habitats in which to lay her eggs. After oviposition the female mosquito takes another blood-meal and after 2–3 days (in the tropics) a further batch of eggs is matured. This process of blood-feeding and egg maturation, followed by oviposition, is repeated several times throughout the female's life and is referred to as the gonotrophic cycle.

Although male mosquitoes have a conspicuous proboscis, their mandibles and maxillae are insufficiently developed for piercing the skin and blood-feeding, instead they feed on the nectar of flowers, and other naturally occurring sugary secretions. Males are consequently unable to transmit any disease to man. Sugar feeding is not, however, restricted to males, females may also feed on sugary substances to obtain energy for flight and dispersal, but only in a few species (the autogenous ones), is this type of food sufficient for egg development.

Oviposition and biology of the eggs

Depending on the species, female mosquitoes lay about 30–300 eggs at any one oviposition. Eggs are brown or blackish. In many Culicinae they are elongate or approximately ovoid in shape while in the Anophelinae they are usually boat-shaped (see Fig. 1.8). Many mosquitoes, such as species of *Anopheles*, *Culex* and some *Mansonia*, lay their eggs directly on the water surface. In *Anopheles* the eggs are laid singly and float on the water, whereas those of *Culex* and some *Mansonia* (subgenus *Coquillettidia*) are laid stuck together in 'egg rafts' which float on the water surface (see Fig. 1.15). None of the eggs of these mosquitoes can survive desiccation and consequently if they become dry they die. In the tropics eggs hatch within about 2–3 days, but in cooler temperate countries they may not hatch until after about 7–14 days, or longer.

Other mosquitoes, such as those belonging to the genera *Aedes* and *Haemagogus*, do not lay their eggs on the water surface but deposit them just above the water line on damp substrates, such as mud and leaf litter or on the inside walls of tree holes and clay pots (see Fig. 1.15). These eggs can withstand desiccation for weeks, months, or even years, and still remain viable and capable of hatching when they are flooded with water. Because the eggs are laid above the water line of breeding places it may be many weeks or months before they are flooded with water, and thus have the opportunity to hatch. However, even when flooded, hatching may be extended over long periods because the eggs hatch in instalments. Moreover, *Aedes* eggs sometimes require repeated immersions in water, followed by short periods of desiccation, before they will hatch. *Aedes* eggs may also enter a quiescent state called diapause, and will not hatch until diapause is terminated (broken). Environmental stimuli, such as a reduction in oxygen content of the water or changes in daylength often break diapause. In temperate regions many *Aedes* species overwinter as diapausing eggs.

Larval biology

Mosquito larvae can be distinguished from all other aquatic insects by being legless and having a bulbous thorax that is wider than both the head and abdomen. There are four active larval instars. All mosquito larvae require water in which to develop; no mosquito has larvae that can withstand desiccation although they may be able to survive short periods amongst, for example, wet mud.

Mosquito larvae have a well developed head, bearing a pair of antennae and a pair of compound eyes. Prominent mouth brushes are present in most species and serve to sweep water containing minute food particles into the mouth. The thorax is roundish in outline and has various simple and branched hairs which are usually long and conspicuous. The segmented abdomen has nine visible segments, most of which have simple or branched hairs (see Figs. 1.9 and 1.16). The last segment has two paired groups of long hairs forming the caudal setae, and a larger group of hairs forming the ventral brush (see Figs. 1.10 and 1.16), and ends in two pairs of transparent, sausage-shaped gills. Although called gills they are not concerned with osmoregulation but with respiration.

Mosquito larvae, with the exception of *Mansonia* species (and a few other mosquito species), must come to the water surface to breathe. Atmospheric air is taken in through a pair of spiracles situated dorsally on the eighth abdominal segment. In the subfamilies Toxorhynchitinae and Culicinae these spiracles are situated at the end of a single dark-coloured and heavily sclerotised tube termed the siphon (see Fig. 1.16). *Mansonia* larvae possess a specialised siphon that is more or less conical, pointed at the tip and supplied with prehensile hairs and serrated cutting structures (see Fig. 3.10). These enable the siphon to be inserted into the roots or stems of aquatic plants and thus oxygen for larval respiration is obtained from the plants. In contrast larvae of the Anophelinae do not have siphons (see Figs. 1.10 and 1.13).

Mosquito larvae feed on yeasts, bacteria, protozoa and numerous other plant and animal micro-organisms found in the water. Some, such as *Anopheles* species are surface feeders, whereas many others browse over the bottom of habitats. A few mosquitoes are carnivorous or cannibalistic. There are four larval instars and in tropical countries larval development, that is the time from egg hatching to pupation, can be as short as 5–7 days, but many species require about 7–14 days. In temperate areas the larval period may last several weeks or months, and several species overwinter as larvae.

Larval habitats

Mosquito larval habitats vary from large and usually permanent collections of water, such as fresh water swamps, marshes, rice fields and borrow pits to smaller collections of temporary water such as small pools, puddles, water-filled car tracks, ditches, drains and gulleys. A variety of 'natural container habitats' also provide breeding places, such as water-filled tree holes, rock pools, water-filled bamboo stumps, bromeliads, pitcher plants, leaf axils in banana, pineapple and other plants, water-filled split coconut husks and snail shells. Larvae also occur in wells and 'man-made container habitats', such as clay pots, water-storage jars, tin cans, discarded kitchen utensils and motor vehicle tyres. Some species prefer shaded larval habitats while others like sunlit habitats. Many species cannot survive in water polluted with organic debris whereas others can breed prolifically in water contaminated with excreta or rotting vegetables and plants. A few mosquitoes breed almost exclusively in brackish or salt water, such as in salt water marshes and mangrove swamps, and are consequently restricted to mostly coastal areas. Some species are less specific in their requirements and can tolerate a wide range of different types of breeding places.

Almost any collection of permanent or temporary water can constitute a mosquito larval habitat, but larvae are usually absent from large expanses of uninterrupted water such as lakes, especially if they have large numbers of fish and other predators which are likely to eat mosquito larvae. They are also usually absent from large rivers and fast flowing waters, except that they may occur in marshy areas and isolated pools and puddles formed at the edges of flowing water.

Pupal biology

All mosquito pupae are aquatic and comma-shaped. The head and thorax are combined to form the cephalothorax which has a pair of respiratory trumpets dorsally (Fig. 1.6). The segmented abdomen has numerous short hairs and the last segment terminates in a pair of oval and flattened structures termed the paddles (see Figs. 1.11 and 1.18). Some of the developing structures of the adult mosquito can be seen through the integument of the cephalothorax, the most conspicuous features being a pair of dark compound eyes, folded wings, legs and the proboscis (Fig. 1.6).

Pupae do not feed but spend most of their time at the water surface taking in air through the respiratory trumpets. If disturbed they swim up and down in the water in a jerky fashion.

Pupae of *Mansonia* differ in that they have relatively long breathing trumpets, which are modified to enable them to pierce

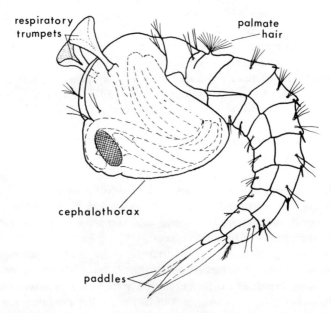

Fig. 1.6 *Anopheles* pupa.

aquatic vegetation and obtain their oxygen in a similar fashion to the larvae (see Fig. 3.10). As a consequence *Mansonia* pupae remain submerged and rarely come to the water surface.

In the tropics the pupal period in mosquitoes lasts only 2–3 days but in cooler temperate regions pupal development may be extended over 9–12 days, or longer. At the end of pupal life the skin on the dorsal surface of the cephalothorax splits, and the adult mosquito struggles out.

Adult biology and behaviour

As already mentioned (p. 6), females of most species of mosquito require a blood-meal, either before or more usually after mating, before the eggs can develop. Many species bite man to obtain their blood-meals and a few may feed on man in preference to any other animals. However, others prefer feeding on non-human animals and many never bite man. Species that usually bite man are said to be anthropophagic in their feeding habits, while those that feed mainly on other animals are called zoophagic. Mosquitoes that feed on birds are sometimes called ornithophagic instead of zoophagic. Females are attracted to hosts by various stimuli emanating from them, such as body odours, carbon dioxide and heat. Vision usually plays only a minor role in host orientation but some species are attracted by the silhouette or movement of their hosts. Some species feed more or less indiscriminately at any time of the day or night, others are mainly diurnal or nocturnal in their biting habits.

A few species of mosquitoes frequently enter houses to feed on man and are said to be endophagic in their feeding habits, whereas those that bite their hosts outside houses are called exophagic. After having bitten man, or animals, either inside or outside houses, mosquitoes seek resting places in which to shelter during digestion of their blood-meals. Some species rest inside houses during the time required for blood digestion and maturation of the ovaries and are called endophilic. In contrast mosquitoes that rest outdoors are termed exophilic. Female adults of *Aedes aegypti* (a vector of yellow fever), for example, are usually anthropophagic, exophagic and exophilic, whereas adults of *Anopheles gambiae* (African malaria vector) are mainly anthropophagic, endophagic and endophilic. Few mosquitoes, however, are entirely anthropophagic or zoophagic, endophagic or exophagic, endophilic or exophilic. Instead, most show various degrees of these behavioural patterns; in other words all these terms are relative. The feeding behaviour of a species may also change, in certain areas and at certain seasons a species may bite man predominantly (anthropophagic) inside houses (endophagic) and remain in houses afterwards (endophilic), whereas at other times, especially if there are few people but many animals in the area, the species may become predominantly zoophagic, and also exophagic and exophilic. Some species are less adaptable in their feeding behaviour and, will never rest inside houses or enter them to feed on man.

The biting behaviour of female mosquitoes may be very important in the epidemiology of disease transmission. Mosquitoes that feed on man predominantly out of doors and late at night, will not bite many young children because they will be indoors and asleep at this time. Thus, young children will be less likely to be infected with any diseases that these mosquitoes might transmit. During hot and dry periods of the year substantial numbers of people may sleep out of doors and as a consequence be bitten more frequently by exophagic mosquitoes. Some mosquitoes bite predominantly within forests or wooded areas. Consequently, man will only get bitten when he visits these places. Clearly the behaviour of both people and mosquitoes may be relevant in disease transmission.

The resting behaviour of adult mosquitoes may be an important consideration in planning control measures. In many malaria control campaigns the interior surfaces of houses, such as walls and ceilings, are sprayed with residual insecticides, such as DDT, to kill adult mosquitoes resting on them. This approach will, of course, only be effective in controlling malaria if the mosquito vectors are endophilic.

Mosquitoes usually disperse less than 2 km and most only fly a few hundred metres from their breeding places. A few species, principally those inhabiting temperate and cold northern climates, may disperse much further, especially just after emergence. Mosquitoes sometimes get transported long distances by wind.

In tropical countries adult mosquitoes probably live, on average, only about 2–3 weeks, but in temperate climates the average life expectancy may be 4–6 weeks or longer, and species which overwinter as fertilised and hibernating adults live for many months. It seems that males usually have a shorter life–span than females.

CLASSIFICATION OF MOSQUITOES

Subfamily Toxorhynchitinae

This subfamily comprises a single genus, *Toxorhynchites*, which contains about 70, mainly tropical, species.

Adult mosquitoes are large and colourful, being metallic bluish or greenish with orange and red tufts of hairs on some abdominal segments. Adults are easily recognised by the possession of a proboscis that is recurved in both sexes and incapable of piercing the skin to take blood-meals (Fig. 1.7). Consequently since

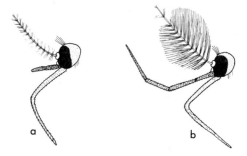

Fig. 1.7   Heads of *Toxorhynchites* adults. (a) Female; (b) male.

neither sex can bite, they are of no medical importance. Their larvae are large, often dark reddish in colour and, like the Culicinae, have a siphon. They are predacious on larvae of other mosquitoes and of their own kind. They have occasionally been introduced into areas in the hope that their predacious habits will help reduce the numbers of pest mosquitoes. They are mainly found in container habitats such as tree holes, pitcher plants, bamboo stumps, tin cans and pots.

Subfamily Anophelinae

Three genera are included in this subfamily but only the genus *Anopheles*, which contains important malaria vectors, is of medical importance. The following characters serve to separate this genus from all the 33 genera of the Culicidae.

Anopheline eggs

Eggs are laid singly on the water surface. In most species they are typically boat-shaped and, laterally, have a pair of floats (Fig. 1.8). Anopheline eggs are unable to withstand desiccation.

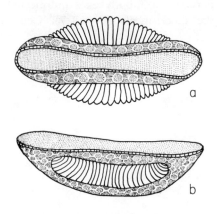

Fig. 1.8 *Anopheles* eggs. (a) Dorsal view; (b) lateral view.

Anopheline larvae

Larvae lack a siphon and lie parallel to the water surface, not subtended at an angle as are the culicines. They are surface feeders and spend most of their time at the water surface. Examination under a microscope shows that the abdomen has small, brown, sclerotised plates, called tergal plates, on the dorsal surface of abdominal tergites 1–8. In addition most or all of these segments have a pair of well developed palmate hairs, sometimes called float hairs (Figs. 1.9 and 1.10). These abdominal palmate hairs

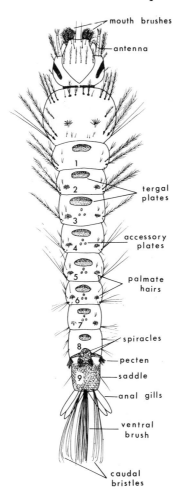

Fig. 1.9 *Anopheles* larva, dorsal view.

and the single pair on the thorax come into contact with the water surface and aid in keeping the larvae parallel to the surface. All these structures identify larvae as belonging to the genus *Anopheles*.

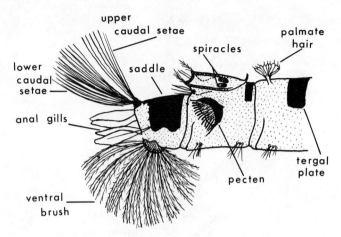

Fig. 1.10   Terminal segments of *Anopheles* larva in lateral view.

Anopheline pupae

The respiratory trumpets are short and broad distally, thus appearing conical (see Figs. 1.6 and 1.11a), whereas in most culicines the trumpets are narrower and more cylindrical. The most reliable characteristic for identifying anopheline pupae is the

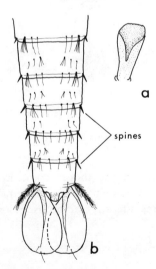

Fig. 1.11   *Anopheles* pupa. (a) Short broad respiratory trumpet; (b) characteristic spines on abdomen.

presence of short, peg-like spines situated laterally near the distal margins of abdominal segments 2–3 or 3–7 (Fig. 1.11b); in the culicines there are no such spines.

Anopheline adults

Adult *Anopheles* usually rest with their bodies at an angle to the surface, that is with proboscis and abdomen in a straight line (see Fig. 1.13). In some species they rest at almost right angles to the surface, whereas in others, such as *An. culicifacies*, the angle is much smaller. This is a very useful characteristic allowing adults resting in houses and elsewhere to be readily identified as *Anopheles*. Most, but not all, *Anopheles* mosquitoes have the dark (usually blackish) and pale (usually whitish or creamy white) scales on the wing veins arranged in 'blocks' or specific areas (Fig. 1.12) forming a distinctive spotted pattern which differs according to species. A few species, however, have the veins covered more or less uniformly with dark (often brown) scales.

The most reliable way to distinguish between adult *Anopheles* and Culicinae is by examination of their heads. The first procedure is to determine the sex of the adults: female mosquitoes have non-plumose antennae while males have plumose antennae. If the adults are females and also *Anopheles* then the palps will be about as long as the proboscis and usually lie closely alongside it (Fig. 1.13). The palps are usually blackish with broad or narrow rings of pale scales, especially on the apical half. In male *Anopheles* the palps are also about as long as the proboscis but are distinctly swollen at the ends and are said to be clubbed (Fig. 1.13), they may also have rings of pale scales apically.

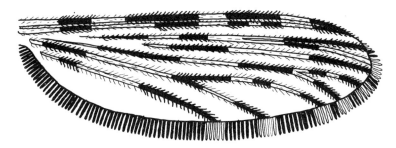

Fig. 1.12 *Anopheles* wing showing arrangement of dark and pale scales on veins arranged in 'blocks'.

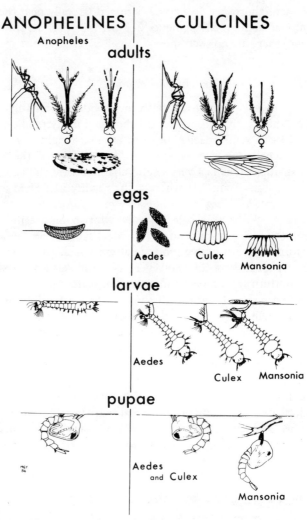

ANOPHELINES | **CULICINES**

Anopheles

adults

♂ ♀ ♂ ♀

eggs

Aedes Culex

Mansonia

larvae

Aedes

Culex Mansonia

pupae

Aedes
and Culex

Mansonia

Fig. 1.13 Diagrammatic representation of the principal characters separating the various stages in the life-cycle of anopheline and culicine mosquitoes.

Other minor differences between *Anopheles* and the Culicinae are that (i) in both sexes of *Anopheles* the scutellum is rounded posteriorly and has setae along the entire edge; (ii) only one spermotheca is present in the females; and (iii) in both sexes the middle lobe of the salivary glands is considerably shorter than the two outer lobes (Fig. 1.14).

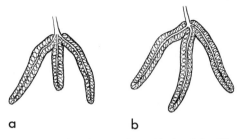

Fig. 1.14 Salivary glands of adult mosquitoes. (a) *Anopheles*; (b) culicine.

The principal characters for separating the various stages in the life-cycles of anopheline and culicine mosquitoes are given in Table 1.1.

Table 1.1 Principal characters distinguishing anopheline and culicine mosquitoes.

Stage	Anophelinae	Culicinae
Eggs	Laid singly, possess floats	Laid singly or in egg rafts or masses. Never possess floats
Larvae	Never have a siphon. Lie parallel to water surface. Have abdominal palmate hairs and tergal plates	All larvae have a short or long siphon. Subtend an angle from the water surface. No palmate hairs or tergal plates
Pupae	Breathing trumpets short and broad apically. Short peg-like abdominal spines on segments 2 or 3 to 7	Breathing trumpet short or long, opening not broad. No spines or abdominal segments 2 to 7
Adults (both sexes)	Rest at an angle to any surface. In most species dark and pale scales on wing veins arranged in distinct 'blocks'	Rest with the bodies more or less parallel to the surface. Scales on wing veins not arranged in 'blocks', scaled frequently all brown or blackish, or a mixture of pale and dark scales scattered on veins
Adult females (non-plumose antennae)	Palps about as long as proboscis	Palps much shorter than proboscis
Adult males (plumose antennae)	Palps about as long as proboscis and swollen at ends	Palps about as long as proboscis, but never swollen at ends, may be hairy distally

Subfamily Culicinae

There are 33 genera in this subfamily and the most important medically are *Aedes, Culex, Mansonia, Haemagogus* and *Sabethes*. The following characters serve to separate the Culicinae from the *Anopheles* mosquitoes. Methods for distinguishing between the more important genera within the Culicinae are given in Chapter 3.

Culicine eggs

Eggs never have floats. They are laid either singly (e.g. *Aedes*) or in the form of egg rafts that float on the water surface (e.g. *Culex* and some *Mansonia*), or are deposited as sticky masses glued to the undersides of floating vegetation (some *Mansonia*) (Fig. 1.15).

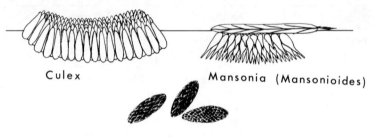

Culex   Mansonia (Mansonioides)

Aedes

Fig. 1.15 Mosquito eggs. *Culex* egg raft floating on water surface, *Mansonia* subgenus (*Mansonioides*) eggs glued to undersurface of floating vegetation, and individual *Aedes* eggs—which are deposited on damp surfaces.

Culicine larvae

All culicine larvae possess a siphon (Fig. 1.16), which may be long or short. They hang upside down at an angle from the water surface when they are getting air (see Fig. 1.13), except for *Mansonia* larvae which insert their specialised siphons into aquatic plants and remain submerged (see Fig. 3.10). There are no abdominal palmate hairs or tergal plates on culicine larvae.

Culicine pupae

The length of the respiratory trumpets is variable, but the trumpets are generally longer, more cylindrical and their openings

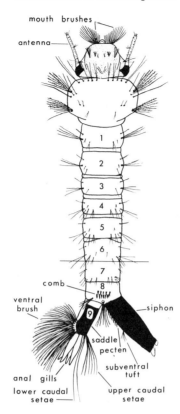

Fig. 1.16 Culicine larva, dorsal view but segments seven to nine are lateral to display important characters.

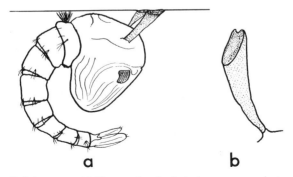

Fig. 1.17 Culicine pupa. (a) Elongated and relatively narrow respiratory trumpet; (b) pupal position at water surface.

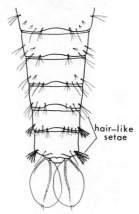

Fig. 1.18 Culicine pupa showing abdominal hair-like setae (note absence of spines).

narrower (Fig. 1.17a) than in *Anopheles*. Abdominal segments 2–7 lack peg-like spines although they have numerous setae (Fig. 1.18).

Culicine adults

In life adults rest with the thorax and abdomen more or less parallel to the surface (Fig. 1.13). The wing veins are commonly covered with scales of a uniform brown or black colour. Sometimes, however, there are contrasting dark and pale scales but they are not arranged in distinctive areas or 'blocks', as found in many *Anopheles* adults.

The most reliable method for identifying the Culicinae is to examine their heads. In females (which have non-plumose antennae), the palps are shorter than the proboscis. In males (which have plumose antennae), the palps are about as long as the proboscis but are not swollen distally and hence do not appear clubbed (see Fig. 1.13). However, they may be turned upwards distally, and in many species they are covered with long hairs so that, superficially, they can appear to be somewhat swollen apically, but more careful inspection shows that the palps in male culicines are not clubbed.

Other minor differences that separate the Culicinae from *Anopheles* are that in culicines the scutellum is trilobed and the scutellar setae are restricted to these lobes. There are 2–3 spermathecae in the females and the middle lobe of the salivary glands is about as long as the outer two lobes (see Fig. 1.14).

MEDICAL IMPORTANCE

Although in many temperate countries mosquitoes may be of little or no importance as disease vectors they can, nevertheless, cause considerable annoyance because of their bites. The greatest numbers of mosquitoes are found in the northern areas of the temperate regions, especially near or within the Arctic Circle where the numbers biting can be so great at certain times of the year as to make almost any outdoor activity impossible. Because of their elongated mouthparts female mosquitoes have little difficulty in biting through clothing such as socks, shirts, trousers and woollen garments, but clothing with a much closer weave of material may prevent this.

Mosquitoes are important as vectors of malaria, various forms of filariasis and numerous arboviruses, the best known being dengue and yellow fever. Their role in the transmission of these diseases is discussed in the next two chapters.

MOSQUITO CONTROL

Greater efforts have been made to control mosquitoes than any other biting insects and a vast literature has accumulated on control operations.

Control measures which are directed against specific vectors, such as *Aedes aegypti*, *Culex quinquefasciatus* and the malaria vectors, are described in more detail in Chapters 2 and 3, only the broader principles of control are outlined here.

Control measures can be directed at either the immature aquatic stages or the adults, or at both stages simultaneously.

Control directed at the immature stages

Biological control

Although often termed naturalist control there is little, if anything, natural about the process. Either the incidence of predators, parasites or pathogens in any habitat must be greatly increased to obtain worthwhile control, or they have to be introduced into habitats from which they were originally absent; such environmental manipulation is not natural. Because biological control methods (biocontrol) do not cause any chemical pollution they are sometimes advocated as a better approach than insecticidal methods. They are, however, usually more difficult to implement and maintain. Moreover, if predators are used it is unlikely that they will prey exclusively on mosquito larvae and pupae but may also eat harmless or beneficial insects. Finally, biological control does not lead to rapid control; it takes some days, or more usually weeks, to cause reductions in mosquito larvae.

Predators
Several attempts have been made to control mosquitoes by using predators. The most commonly used predators are fish. Species of the genera *Gambusia, Poecilia, Sarotherodon* (= *Tilapia*) and *Panchax* have been used, but *G. affinis affinis* and *G. affinis holbrooki*, commonly referred to as 'mosquito fish', have been employed more extensively than any others. Originating in the USA, *Gambusia* has been introduced into the Pacific Islands, Europe, the Middle East, South-east Asia and Africa in attempts to control mosquito larvae.

Some predatory fish can breed in saline waters and can therefore be introduced into salt water habitats. Fish are unsuitable for the control of mosquitoes which breed in small containers, pools and puddles which rapidly dry out. However, some fish such as species of *Nothobranchius* and *Cynolebias*, which are the so called 'instant' or 'annual' fish, have drought resistant eggs and these are more suitable for introducing into small temporary habitats that repeatedly dry out. Polluted waters are also usually unsuitable habitats for most fish, although *Poecilia reticulata* is able to tolerate moderate pollution.

Although fish have sometimes greatly reduced the numbers of larvae in certain habitats, such as borrow pits, ponds and rice fields, they have rarely proved effective in reducing the size of mosquito populations over large areas. Nor is there much convincing evidence that they have significantly decreased the incidence of mosquito-borne diseases.

Other predators of mosquito larvae and pupae include tadpoles of frogs and toads and various aquatic insect larvae, but these have rarely proved effective as control agents. A few mosquitoes have predacious larvae, for example *Toxorhynchites* species. These have been introduced into container habitats in certain areas (e.g. Fiji, Samoa and Hawaii) to control larvae of other container-breeding mosquitoes but results have not been very encouraging.

Pathogens and Parasites

There are numerous pathogens, such as viruses (e.g. iridescent and cytoplasmic polyhedrosis viruses), bacteria (e.g. *Bacillus thuringiensis* var. *israelensis, B. sphaericus*), protozoa (e.g. *Nosema vavraia, Thelohania*) and fungi (e.g. *Coelomomyces, Lagenidium, Culicinomyces*) that cause larval mortality. There are also several parasitic nematodes that kill mosquito larvae and the most promising for control purposes is *Romanomermis culicivorax* which has been commercially mass produced. These parasites and pathogens appear harmless to man.

Although there is considerable interest in biological agents, as yet they cannot be routinely advocated for control, especially in the tropics. The most useful pathogen is *B. thuringiensis* var. *israelensis*, which is easy to mass produce and is formulated as a powder to be sprayed on the water. However, the sprayed formulation is not a live product but consists of dead bacteria that kill mosquito larvae when ingested. It is therefore more of a microbial insecticide than a true biological (living) agent.

Genetic control

Although genetic control methods are directed against the adults rather than the immature stages it is convenient to discuss this strategy here because it is really a form of biological control.

There are several genetic approaches that, at least in theory, can be applied to the control of mosquitoes and other vectors. One technique is to colonise, in the laboratory, large numbers of mosquitoes whose genetic make-up has been altered. For example, genetic manipulation and selective rearing can produce mosquitoes that are refractory to infection with human diseases such as malaria. These insects can be released into the environment in the hope that they may successfully compete with natural populations of susceptible individuals and eventually replace them. Susceptible genes to malaria, for example, will be 'diluted' in the wild population if males genetically normal except for carrying the refractoriness genes, are released in sufficient numbers. It may also be possible to combine refractoriness with insecticide resistance. For example, if populations are sprayed after the release of refractory individuals the refractory adults will survive whereas the natural, non-refractory population will be reduced in size. However, to be effective this approach requires a very close linkage between refractoriness and insecticide-resistance genes. Moreover, if some degree of resistance already exists in the wild population, replacement will not be complete. On the other hand, if there is no resistance in the wild population it might prove difficult to persuade control authorities to allow insecticide resistance genes to be introduced.

Another possibility is the replacement of a vector mosquito with a non-vector species which, in the field, will compete with the vector and eventually replace it. This is known as species replacement. Other methods aim to select genes which cause large distortions in the sex ratio so that excessive numbers of male mosquitoes are produced. Not only are males non-vectors, but introducing a distorted sex ratio gene into populations should lead to reductions in population size.

Sterile-male release techniques involve the production and release into the field of male mosquitoes which are sterile. Sterilisation can be achieved in the laboratory by several methods, such as radiochemical irradiation, use of chemosterilants or production of infertile hybrid males by crossing closely related species. The aim is to introduce sterile males into wild populations to compete with natural fertile males for female mates, and so result in an increased proportion of infertile inseminations. The eggs produced will be sterile and fail to hatch thus causing a reduction, and hopefully the elimination, of the species.

None of these genetic methods is simple and they are usually more difficult to implement than conventional insecticidal measures. There have been a few limited field trials, some of which have shown promise, but genetic control of mosquitoes is still only in the experimental stage. An advantage of genetic methods is that they overcome the increasing problems of insecticide resistance which is fast developing in many mosquito species. There is also no contamination of the environment with insecticides. However, there are difficulties: high technology and expertise are required, and the ability to rear vast numbers of mosquitoes for releasing into the field to compete with, or replace, natural populations. Not all the important vector mosquitoes can be reared in the laboratory, let alone on an enormous scale. Moreover, it is essential that reared mosquitoes live as long and are as healthy and vigorous as wild populations, otherwise they will be unable to compete with them and cause their elimination. Another problem is that changes may evolve in mosquito–parasite relationships so that the parasites (e.g. malaria, filaria), are able to develop in strains of mosquitoes that were originally selected for their refractoriness to infection.

Physical (mechanical or environmental) control

Filling in, source reduction and drainage

A simple form of control consists of filling in, and thus completely eradicating, breeding places. Larval habitats ranging in size from water-filled tree holes to ponds and small marshes can be filled in with rubble, earth, sand, etc. Certain container habitats such as abandoned cans, metal drums, canoes, pots and tyres can be removed and the breeding sources greatly reduced or eliminated. Mosquito breeding in containers which are used to collect and maintain drinking water, such as water-storage jars and village pots, could be reduced by covering up their openings, but this is seldom very popular with the owners and the practice becomes neglected. In some areas the introduction of a reliable piped water supply should help reduce the dependence on water-storage containers and thereby reduce breeding of species such as *Aedes aegypti*. Some mosquitoes breed in septic tanks, faulty soak-away pits, large water-storage tanks and cisterns, but this type of breeding can be prevented if existing covers are repaired or new ones fitted.

Larval breeding places such as ponds, borrow pits, fresh and salt water marshes can be drained. An important advantage of filling in, draining or removing larval habitats is that such measures can lead to permanent control, but this approach is not always feasible. It is impossible, for example, to fill in all the scattered, small and temporary collections of water such as pools, vehicle tracks and puddles which may appear during the rainy season. Larger and more permanent habitats such as swamps may prove too costly to drain. Moreover, the local people may, understandably, not want certain breeding places such as rice fields, ponds which may be used as fish farms, and borrow pits providing drinking water for man and his livestock, to be either drained or filled in: such habitats are an essential part of life. The feasibility of eradicating breeding places must be assessed individually in each area.

Habitat changes

If it is impossible to eliminate aquatic habitats, it may be possible to alter them to make them unsuitable for mosquito breeding. For example, many mosquitoes breed in small and more or less isolated pools, or in marshy areas that commonly form at the edges of streams, especially when these have a twisting and winding course. By straightening and steepening the banks of streams and possibly altering their course to prevent the formation of small pools, breeding can be greatly reduced.

Shallow ponds that have sloping edges and a fluctuating water level, resulting in exposed muddy areas, provide ideal breeding sites for many *Aedes* mosquitoes which lay their eggs not on the water surface but on exposed muddy and waterlogged soil. Mosquito breeding can be prevented in these habitats by changing the sloping shore line to one that has well demarcated and steep, almost vertical, banks. Although the water level may still fluctuate it will no longer expose large marshy and muddy areas. Consequently, breeding by *Aedes* mosquitoes will be greatly reduced, or even eliminated.

Cutting down overhanging vegetation to increase sunlight on the water may prevent breeding by species that like shaded habitats, whereas planting vegetation near water may stop breeding by sun-loving species. Similarly, the removal of rooted or floating vegetation may result in reducing mosquito breeding, especially by species of *Mansonia* which require plants to obtain their oxygen requirements. On the other hand, the presence of a dense coverage of vegetation can prevent breeding by species that prefer exposed water surfaces.

Impoundments

Instead of draining marshy areas they can be excavated to form areas of deep water with well defined vertical banks. This process is called impoundment. It completely alters the habitat and makes it unsuitable for mosquitoes which were previously breeding in either numerous small pools scattered over extensive marshy areas or in larger expanses of shallow water with dense growths of vegetation. Both small and large, fresh and salt water, marshy areas can be converted to impounded waters.

Whenever an aquatic habitat is not eliminated, but modified to prevent breeding of certain mosquitoes, there is the danger that such environmental changes will favour the breeding of other species that were previously either absent, or present in only small numbers.

Chemical control

Paris green

One of the earlier chemicals used to prevent mosquito breeding was Paris green (a copper aceto-arsenite), which was applied to the water surface as a very fine dust. After ingestion by mosquito larvae during filter feeding it acted mainly as a stomach poison. It was particularly effective against surface feeding mosquitoes such as *Anopheles*. More recently Paris green has been incorporated into small granules of vermiculite or bentonite which float on the water surface, and also into small sand pellets which sink to the bottom. This latter formulation is particularly effective against mosquito larvae that feed on the bottom. Granular and pellet formulations are better at penetrating dense covers of aquatic vegetation than dusts and are therefore more suited to habitats with vegetation.

Oils

Another method of controlling mosquito larvae is by the application of mineral oils to the water surface. Originally diesel oils, fuel oils or kerosene (paraffin), were sprayed on to water. Larvae are killed not so much by the oils physically blocking their tracheae and suffocating them, but by a combination of the fumigant effects of the oils toxic aromatic hydrocarbons and by the more stable fraction interfering with air intake at the water surface. Because of the poor spreading power of these oils about 300–500 $l\,ha^{-1}$ of oil are needed. Specially prepared commercial oils (for example Flit MLO, ARCO larvicide, Malariol HS), containing spreading agents have been introduced, which have much better spreading powers so that only about 50–100 or even 10–20 $l\,ha^{-1}$ are needed.

Larval habitats have to be treated with chemicals, such as Paris green or oils, about every 7–10 days in most tropical countries to ensure that larvae hatching from eggs are killed before they pupate and give rise to adults. Less frequent applications can be made in cooler temperate areas because the speed of development of the immature stages of mosquitoes is much slower.

Residual insecticides

The advent, in the 1940s, of residual organochlorine insecticides such as DDT, HCH and dieldrin, and later the organophosphate and carbamate insecticides, ushered in a new phase of mosquito control. The use of Paris green and oils was more or less abandoned because much better control was achieved by spraying breeding places with these insecticides.

A set-back in the use of organochlorine larvicides is the development by some mosquitoes of insecticide resistance. Another difficulty is their extreme persistence in the soil and in animal and plant tissues which makes them biological pollutants. The World Health Organisation no longer recommends their use as mosquito larvicides. In their place, the less persistent and biodegradable organophosphate and carbamate insecticides are now recommended to kill mosquito larvae. The organochlorines, however, can still be used for residual spraying of houses (pp. 56–57 in Chapter 2).

The insecticides most commonly used for controlling mosquito larvae include organophosphates such as temephos (Abate), fenthion (Baytex), malathion and chlorpyrifos (Dursban). Dursban is more toxic to most larvae than Abate but causes higher mortalities amongst fish and other aquatic life, and is consequently not so widely used.

Application procedures

Liquid formulations do not easily penetrate dense growths of aquatic vegetation, better penetration is achieved if insecticides are applied as granules or pellets. Some granules are formulated to sink to the bottom of breeding places, whereas others float on the water surface, and some are made for rapid release of toxicants, others for a slower release. Gelatin capsules containing oil solutions of insecticides are also available. They float on the water surface and the gelatin envelope dissolves to release its insecticidal contents.

Insecticides for larval control are often sprayed from knapsack-type sprayers carried on the back of operators, but they can also be dispersed from various insecticidal spraying machines mounted on the back of landrovers or other suitable vehicles. Sometimes, especially if large and/or inaccessible areas require spraying, aerial applications are made from helicopters or light aircraft.

The dosage rate per hectare varies according to the insecticide, the mosquito species and the method of application. For example, ground application rates are usually two-to-four times greater than aerial applications because the former methods do not give such good coverage. Dosage rates usually have to be increased if the water is highly polluted or contains substantial amounts of vegetation.

Although organochlorine, organophosphate and carbamate insecticides are known as residual insecticides they have very little residual effect when used as mosquito larvicides. Consequently, they must be sprayed on larval habitats about as frequently as oils, i.e. every 7–10 days in most tropical areas.

Eggs and pupae
Most insecticides will not kill mosquito eggs, nor will their presence in the water deter gravid females from ovipositing. Relatively few insecticides are very efficient at killing mosquito pupae. Chemical control measures against the immature stages of mosquitoes are mainly directed at killing larvae.

Integrated control

It has become fashionable to advocate integrated control, which usually means combining biological and insecticidal methods. For example, the introduction of predacious fish to breeding places which are also sprayed with insecticides that have minimum effect on the fish. However, it is better to regard integrated control as any approach that takes into consideration more than one method, whether these are directed at only the larvae or adults, or both.

Control directed at adults

Personal protection

Much can be done to reduce the likelihood of being bitten by mosquitoes. Houses, hospitals and other buildings can have windows, doors and ventilators covered with mosquito screening, made either of strong plastic or non-corrosive metal. It is essential that screening is kept in good repair. Screens with 6–8 meshes per centimetre will exclude most mosquitoes. Finer mesh screening will keep out smaller biting flies, some of which may be vectors, but it will appreciably reduce ventilation and light. Screening in most cases need only be extended to about the third floor of buildings because few mosquitoes will fly higher than this to enter buildings. If houses are unscreened, or if screening is defective, mosquito nets with 9–10 meshes per centimetre can be used. These should be tucked in under the mattress or bedding never allowed to drape loosely over the bed; torn nets are useless unless they have been impregnated with a persistent pyrethroid insecticide like permethrin, then even torn nets are useful. Nets should be placed over beds before sunset. The main disadvantage of nets is that they reduce ventilation.

Small spray guns (e.g. 'Flit-guns') filled either with pyrethrum dissolved in kerosene, or some other knock-down insecticide, can be used early each evening in rooms to kill resting mosquitoes that may later try to bite the occupants. Small aerosol canisters containing a fast-acting knock-down insecticide are sold widely for killing houseflies and other obnoxious insects including mosquitoes. When used properly they can be an effective, but costly, method of protection.

Suitable insect repellents in the form of oils, creams or aerosols, can provide temporary protection. The best commercially available repellents usually contain diethytoluamide (DET) or dimethyl phthalate (DMP). Repellents are normally applied to exposed areas of skin, such as wrists, arms, hands, neck and face taking care to avoid the eyes where severe irritation and inflammation may occur. They should also be applied to the ankles even if socks are worn. Mosquitoes are not usually deterred from biting through clothing. To prevent this, clothing may be lightly sprayed with suitable repellents such as diethyltoluamide. Normally, repellents remain effective for only about 2 hours, but clothing specially impregnated with repellents may remain effective for several weeks or even months.

Aerosols, mists and fogs

Oil solutions or emulsions of insecticides can be introduced into a cold high velocity air stream generated by spraying machines to produce mists, fogs or aerosols of insecticide. Alternatively, insecticidal oils can be introduced into specially heated chambers, or into the hot exhaust fumes of spraying machines, for vaporisation and the production of thermal fogs or aerosols. Usually the term mist is applied to formulations that are composed of droplets with a volume median diameter (vmd) of about 50–100 μm, while aerosols and fogs consist of droplets with a vmd of less than 50 μm. The term 'vmd' refers to the median droplet size of a spray, in other words one half of the volume of the spray is composed of droplets larger than this, while the other half consists of smaller droplets.

Fogging and aerosol producing machines can be mounted on vehicles or on aeroplanes and helicopters. Insecticidal mists or fogs are usually used to kill adult mosquitoes, especially those resting in vegetation or other areas that cannot be reached by more conventional methods. Indoor resting adults may sometimes be killed by this method.

Several different insecticides can be used in fogging, including malathion and synthetic pyrethroids. Whatever insecticide is used there is very little residual effect. Consequently, although resting mosquitoes are killed, the sprayed area may become rapidly reinvaded by mosquitoes flying in from adjacent areas, or by newly emerged individuals originating from breeding sites within the area. Therefore, repetitive applications may be needed before the mosquitoes in an area are controlled. Aerosol applications are often combined with other control measures, such as larviciding and the spraying of houses with residual insecticides.

Ultra-low-volume (ULV) applications
The main bulk of any liquid insecticidal formulation consists of the diluent or solvent; the actual amount of the active insecticide is small. Greater efficiency can be achieved if concentrated insecticidal solutions are sprayed sparsely over an area, than if much larger applications containing the same quantity of insecticide, but dispersed in a large volume of solvent, are used. An insecticidal tank, on a vehicle or aeroplane, filled with concentrated insecticide solution can spray much larger areas before refilling than if it contained more conventional formulations. This technique, when very small droplets forming a fog or aerosol of concentrated insecticide are produced, is known as ultra-low-volume (ULV) spraying. Whereas a standard rate of application of an insecticide solution might be 5–28 l ha^{-1}, ULV application will be only about 0·074–1·1 l ha^{-1}.

With aerial applications the droplet size of the insecticide leaving the aeroplane should be bigger (150–200 μm) than for ground-based applications (50–100 μm), because the droplets decrease in size as they fall to the ground, due to evaporation. The height at which spraying is undertaken will also determine optimum droplet size. Small droplets are generally required to kill adult mosquitoes because it is desirable to maintain a dense cloud of droplets in the air near the ground to kill resting and flying individuals. Occasionally ULV methods are used for larviciding, and then larger droplets (150–250 μm) are required so that they fall as rapidly as possible on the water.

ULV techniques are more applicable to insecticides with low volatility and high specific gravity because these characteristics will tend to reduce losses due to drift and evaporation. Malathion is a suitable insecticide and is often used in ULV applications, others include fenthion (Baytex), chlorpyrifos (Dursban) and naled (Dibrom), also synthetic and natural pyrethrums.

Applications of aerosols and fogs are best made in calm weather, and usually in the late evenings or early mornings when there are usually fewer thermals rising from the ground and less turbulence. Local conditions of terrain and climate as well as application techniques and type of insecticides will dictate the timing and exact operational procedures.

Usually there is little residual effect from ULV applications, but concentrates of temephos (Abate) have given good control of *Aedes aegypti* for several weeks.

Residual house-spraying

Some mosquitoes, such as many but not all malaria vectors, *Culex quinquefasciatus* and some *Mansonia* species rest inside houses or man-made animal shelters before and/or after blood-feeding. This knowledge prompted the widespread adoption in malaria campaigns of spraying the interior surfaces of walls and roofs of houses, and sometimes animal shelters, with residual insecticides such as DDT. The whitish powder of insecticide that is deposited on these surfaces kills mosquitoes that rest on them. For greater details of this method see the section on control in Chapter 2.

Dichlorvos strips

Strips of polyvinyl-chloride plastic, impregnated with the fumigant organophosphate insecticide dichlorvos (DDVP), are sold in many countries for killing household insects such as houseflies and mosquitoes. Their effectiveness depends on the build-up of a minimum concentration of fumigant (about $0.1 \mu g l^{-1}$ air). Consequently the number of strips per room depends on its size. A single 5×25 cm strip is required per $28 m^3$ of space, and will probably give a high kill of mosquitoes for 8–10 weeks. They are not very effective in houses or rooms with a lot of ventilation, and should not be used in rooms in which infants, old people or those with bronchial complaints are confined. Although under certain conditions they can be useful in killing household insects, they have not proved effective on a large scale in controlling house-frequenting (endophilic) mosquitoes.

Chapter 2
Anopheline Mosquitoes

The subfamily Anophelinae contains three genera, but as explained in the previous chapter only the genus *Anopheles* is of any medical importance. *Anopheles* mosquitoes have a world-wide distribution, occurring not only in tropical areas but also in temperate regions. There are about 380 different species. The most important disease carried by *Anopheles* mosquitoes is malaria. Some *Anopheles* species are also vectors of filariasis, especially that caused by *Wuchereria bancrofti*, and a few also transmit *Brugia malayi* and *Brugia timori*. Certain species also transmit arboviruses.

EXTERNAL MORPHOLOGY OF *ANOPHELES*

The main features distinguishing adults of the Anophelinae, and in particular the genus *Anopheles*, from other mosquitoes have been given in the previous chapter, but a brief summary is presented here.

Most, but not all, *Anopheles* have spotted wings, that is the dark and pale scales are arranged in small blocks or areas on the veins (see Fig. 1.12). The number, length and arrangement of these dark and pale areas differ considerably in different species and provide useful characters for species identification. Unlike Culicinae the dorsal and ventral surfaces of the abdomen are almost, or entirely, devoid of appressed scales. In both sexes the palps are about as long as the proboscis and in males, but not females, they are enlarged (that is clubbed) apically (see Fig. 1.13).

LIFE-CYCLE OF *ANOPHELES*

After mating and blood-feeding *Anopheles* lay some 50–200 small brown or blackish, boat-shaped eggs (see Fig. 1.8) on the water surface. In most *Anopheles* there is a pair of conspicuous lateral, air-filled chambers called the floats on the eggs, which in a few species extend completely round the egg. These floats help to keep the eggs floating on the water surface. *Anopheles* eggs cannot withstand desiccation and in tropical countries they hatch within 2–3 days, but in colder temperate climates hatching may not occur until after about 2–3 weeks, the duration depending on temperature.

Anopheles larvae have a dark brown or blackish sclerotised head, a roundish thorax with numerous simple and branched hairs and a single pair of thoracic palmate hairs. Six or seven abdominal segments usually have a pair of palmate hairs dorsally (see Fig. 1.9 and 1.10), which help maintain the larvae in a horizontal position at the water surface (see Fig. 1.13). Segments 1–8 have a median sclerotised light or dark brown structure called the tergal plate, which varies in size and shape in different species. In addition each segment may possess one to two very small accessory tergal plates posterior to the main one (see Fig. 1.9). Paired spiracles are present dorsally on the posterior end of the 8th visible segment; there is no siphon. On each side, just below and lateral to the spiracles, is a sclerotised structure bearing teeth, somewhat resembling a comb and called the pecten (see Fig. 1.10). At the end of the last abdominal segment are four sausage-shaped transparent gills which, despite their name, are not used for respiration but have an osmoregulatory function.

As in all mosquitoes there are four larval instars. *Anopheles* larvae are filter feeders and unless disturbed remain at the water surface, feeding on bacteria, yeasts, protozoa and other microorganisms, and also breathing in air through their spiracles. When feeding, larvae rotate their heads through 180° so that the ventrally positioned mouth brushes can sweep the underside of the water surface. Larvae are easily disturbed by shadows or vibrations and respond by swimming quickly to the bottom of the water, they resurface some seconds or minutes afterwards.

Anopheles larvae occur in many different types of large and more or less permanent habitats, ranging from fresh and salt water marshes, mangrove swamps, grassy ditches, rice fields, edges of streams and rivers to ponds and borrow pits. They are also found in small and often temporary breeding places like puddles, hoof prints, wells, discarded tins and sometimes in water-storage pots. A few species occur in water-filled tree holes. In the

Neotropical region (Central and South America and the West Indies) a few *Anopheles* breed in water that collects in the leaf axils of epiphytic plants growing on tree branches, such as bromeliads, which somewhat resemble pineapple plants. Some *Anopheles* prefer habitats with aquatic vegetation, others favour habitats without vegetation, some species like exposed sunlit waters while others prefer more shaded breeding places. In general *Anopheles* prefer clean and unpolluted waters and are usually absent from habitats that contain rotting plants or are contaminated with faeces.

In tropical countries the larval period frequently lasts only about 7 days, but in cooler climates the larval period may be about 2–4 weeks. In temperate areas some *Anopheles* overwinter as larvae and consequently may live many months.

In the comma-shaped pupa the head and thorax are combined to form the cephalothorax, which has a pair of short, trumpet-shaped breathing tubes, situated dorsally, with broad openings (see Fig. 1.6). The abdominal segments have numerous short setae, and segments 2 or 3–7 have, in addition, distinct short, peg-like spines. The last segment terminates in a pair of oval paddles (see Fig. 1.11).

Pupae normally remain floating at the water surface with the aid of the pair of palmate hairs on the cephalothorax, but when disturbed they swim vigorously down to the bottom with characteristic jerky movements. The pupal period lasts 2–3 days in tropical countries but sometimes as long as 1–2 weeks in cooler climates.

Adult biology and behaviour

Most *Anopheles* are crepuscular or nocturnal in their activities. Thus blood-feeding and oviposition normally occur in the evenings, at night or in the early morning around sunrise. Some species such as *An. albimanus*, a malaria vector in Central and South America, bite man mainly outdoors (exophagic) from about sunset to 21.00 hours. In contrast, in Africa species of the *An. gambiae* complex, which contains probably the world's most efficient malaria vectors, bite mainly after 23.00 hours and mostly indoors (endophagic). As already discussed in Chapter 1, the times of biting, and whether adult mosquitoes are exophagic or endophagic, may be important in the epidemiology of diseases.

Both before and after blood-feeding some species will rest in houses (endophilic), whereas others will rest outdoors (exophilic) in a variety of natural shelters, such as amongst vegetation, in rodent burrows, in cracks and crevices in trees, under bridges, in termite mounds, in caves and amongst rock fissures, and cracks in the ground. Most *Anopheles* species are not exclusively exophagic or endophagic, exophilic or endophilic, but exhibit a mixture of these extremes of behaviour. Similarly, few *Anopheles* feed exclusively on either man or non-humans, most feed on both man and animals but the degree of anthropophagism and zoophagism varies according to species. For example, *An. culicifacies*, an important Indian malaria vector, commonly feeds on cattle as well as man, whereas in Africa *An. gambiae sensu stricto* (of the *gambiae* complex) feeds more rarely on cattle and thus maintains a stronger mosquito–man contact. This is one of the reasons why *An. gambiae* is a more efficient malaria vector than *An. culicifacies*.

MEDICAL IMPORTANCE

Biting nuisance

In some areas, although *Anopheles* mosquitoes may not be vectors of any disease they may constitute a biting problem. Usually, however, mosquitoes that cause a biting nuisance, but do not transmit diseases, are various culicines such as *Aedes* species, not anophelines.

Malaria

Anopheles are the most notorious of all vectors of disease to man. Only mosquitoes of the genus *Anopheles* can transmit *Plasmodium* species causing malaria in man, namely *P. falciparum* (malignant tertian), *P. vivax* (benign tertian), *P. malariae* (quartan malaria) and *P. ovale* (ovale benign tertian). Because the sexual cycle of the malaria parasite occurs in the *Anopheles* vector, it is conventional to call the mosquito the definite host, and man the intermediate one.

Male and female malaria gametocytes are ingested by female mosquitoes during blood-feeding on man. They pass to the mosquito's stomach where they undergo cyclical development that

includes a sexual cycle termed sporogony. Only gametocytes survive in the mosquito's stomach, all other blood forms of the malaria
parasites (the asexual forms) are destroyed. Male gametocytes
(microgametocytes) extrude flagella which are the male gametes
(microgametes), and the process is called exflagellation. The microgametes break free and fertilise the female gametes (macroga-
metes) which have formed from the macrogametocytes. As a result of fertilisation a zygote is formed, which elongates to become
an ookinete. This penetrates the wall of the mosquito's stomach
and reaches its outer membrane where it becomes spherical and
develops into an oocyst. The nucleus of the oocyst divides repeatedly to produce numerous spindle-shaped sporozoites. When
the oocyst is fully grown (about 60–80 μm) it ruptures and thousands of sporozoites are released into the haemocele of the mosquito. The sporozoites are carried in the insect's haemolymph
to all parts of the body but most penetrate the salivary glands.
The mosquito is now infective and sporozoites are inoculated into
man the next time the mosquito bites. It has been estimated that
there may be some 70 000 sporozoites in the salivary glands of a
vector.

Oocysts can be seen on the stomach walls of vectors about 4
days after an infective blood-meal; after about 8 days they are
fully grown and rupture. Sporozoites are usually found in the
salivary glands after 9–12 days but the time required for this
cyclical development (exogenous or extrinsic cycle), depends on
both temperature and *Plasmodium* species. For example, at 24°C
sporogony in *P. vivax* takes only 9 days, in *P. falciparum* 11 days,
in *P. malariae* 21 days; at 26°C sporogony of *P. ovale* is completed
in 15 days.

The sporozoite rate, that is the percentage of female vectors
with sporozoites in the salivary glands, varies considerably, not
only from species to species of mosquitoes but also according to
locality and season. Sporozoite rates are often about 1–5 per cent
in species such as *An. gambiae* and *An. arabiensis* of the *An.
gambiae* complex, but less than 1 per cent in many other species
such as *An. albimanus* and *An. culcifacies*. For practical purposes
it can be said that once a vector becomes infective it remains so
throughout its life, although it has not been established that this
is so for all vector–*Plasmodium* combinations.

Malaria formerly occurred in parts of the southern USA and
in many areas of Europe, but due to changes in agricultural prac-

tices, life-style and also control measures, malaria was eradicated from these areas. However, it should be remembered these areas were at the periphery of malaria distribution so it was probably not so difficult to get rid of the disease. During the early 1960s the incidence of malaria was greatly reduced in some tropical countries such as India and Sri Lanka, but for various reasons, including insecticide resistance, bad surveillance, poorly trained and supervised personnel, lack of money and unusual weather, malaria outbreaks recurred in both countries during the late 1960s. The situation in the 1970s deteriorated even further. In other areas such as Africa there has, as yet, been little or no impact on malaria transmission.

Important malaria vectors

Notes are given below on the principal larval habitats and biting behaviour of adults of some of the more important malaria vectors. In such brief notes it is impossible to list all the countries in which the vectors occur, and moreover, their importance as vectors and their behaviour may differ in different areas of their distribution. These notes are no more than a guide. For greater detail of the behaviour and importance of *Anopheles* as malaria vectors in different countries other reference works and books should be consulted.

Malaria vectors of Mexico and Central America

An. albimanus
Texas and Florida in the USA through Central America to Colombia, Ecuador, Venezuela and the Antilles. Larvae in fresh or brackish waters such as pools, puddles, marshes, ponds and lagoons especially those containing floating or grassy vegetation. Prefers sunlight, feeds on man and domestic animals both indoors and outdoors, after feeding adults rest mainly outdoors.

An. albitarsis
Central America to South America and Trinidad. Larvae nearly always in sunlit ponds, large pools and marshes with filamentous algae. Bites man and domestic animals almost indiscriminately, outdoors and also indoors, usually rests outdoors after feeding.

An. aquasalis
Lesser Antilles, Trinidad, Tobago and other nearby islands, Central America to northern parts of Brazil. Tidal salt water marshes, lagoons, salt water regions of rivers, estuaries, rarely fresh water. Sunlit or shaded habitats. Bites man and domestic animals, indoors or outdoors, rests mainly outdoors.

An. aztecus
Mexico at heights of 1500–2200 m. Pools, ponds, lakes, especially with vegetation, canals and even polluted waters. Bites man indoors and outdoors, rests mainly outdoors after feeding.

An. darlingi
Mexico through Central America to Argentina and Chile. Fresh water marshes, lagoons, rice fields, swamps, lakes and ponds, pools and edges of streams, especially with vegetation. Mainly shaded habitats. Feeds mainly on man indoors, remains indoors after feeding.

An. punctimacula
Mexico through Central America to Peru, Brazil, Argentina and Trinidad. Small pools, swamps, grassy pools at edges of streams, prefers shade. Bites man and domestic animals both indoors and outdoors, rests indoors or outdoors after feeding.

Malaria vectors of South America

An. albimanus
See Central America.

An. albitarsis
See Central America.

An. aquasalis
See Central America.

An. bellator
Trinidad, Venezuela, Surinam, Guyana and Brazil. Larvae occur only in water collected in leaf axils of bromeliads, which are epiphytes on trees, prefers partially shaded habitats. Bites man

during daytime in shaded forests, also at night, and may enter houses. Rests indoors after feeding. Although man is favoured host also bites domestic animals.

An. cruzii
Costa Rica, Panama, Ecuador, Bolivia, Colombia, Peru, Brazil and Venezuela. Larvae occur in water collected in leaf axils of bromeliads, partial shade preferred. Bites man indoors and out-doors and after feeding rests indoors or outdoors. It is of main importance as a malaria vector in coastal areas of Brazil.

An. darlingi
See Central America.

An. nuneztovari
Guyana, Venezuela, Colombia, Brazil and Bolivia. Larvae occur in muddy waters of pools, vehicle tracks, hoof prints and small ponds, especially in and around towns, they prefer sunlight. Feeds mainly on animals, but also bites man outdoors and rests outdoors after feeding. Can be an important vector in Colombia and Venezuela.

An. pseudopunctipennis
Antilles, southern USA to Argentina. Pools, puddles, seepage waters and edges of streams, especially habitats with algae. Prefers sunlight. Feeds almost indiscriminately on man and domestic animals, indoors or outdoors, rests outdoors after feeding.

An. punctimacula
See Central America.

Malaria vectors of Africa south of the Sahara

An. gambiae complex
Consists of six very similar species, separated by banding patterns of their polytene chromosomes. They differ in certain aspects of their biology and behaviour.

An. gambiae (formerly called species A of the *gambiae* complex) is widespread in nearly all African countries south of the Sahara and is probably the world's most efficient malaria vector. Larvae occur mainly in temporary habitats such as pools, puddles, hoof prints and borrow pits, but also rice fields. Bites man both indoors and outdoors, in some areas also feeds on domestic animals, rests predominantly indoors after feeding, but may rest outdoors.

An. arabiensis (formerly species B of the *gambiae* complex) is also widespread in most African countries but seems to prefer rather drier savanna areas. Larval habitats are the same as those of *An. gambiae*. Adults bite man and animals, indoors and outdoors, and afterwards rest indoors or outdoors. This species has a greater tendency than *An. gambiae* to bite animals and rest outdoors. An important malaria vector, but generally not so efficient as *An. gambiae*.

An. quadriannulatus (formerly species C of the *gambiae* complex) occurs in Ethiopia, Zanzibar, Zimbabwe, Zambia, Mozambique and southern Africa. As it mainly feeds on cattle, it is not considered an important malaria vector.

An. bwambae (formerly species D of the *An. gambiae* complex) is known from mineral springs in the Semliki forest of Uganda. It is a rare species and is not considered an important malaria vector, though it can transmit malaria within its very restricted range.

An. melas is a salt water breeding species of the *gambiae* complex, it occurs along the coast of West Africa to Congo. Very common in lagoons and mangrove swamps, does not breed in fresh water. Adults behave similarly to *An. gambiae* and are malaria vectors in many coastal areas.

An. merus is the East African equivalent of *An. melas*, it breeds in salt water lagoons and swamps along the coast of East Africa. Biting behaviour of adults is similar to that of *An. gambiae*. It can be a vector in certain coastal areas.

An. funestus
Widespread in Africa south of the Sahara. The most important vector after *An. gambiae* and *An. arabiensis* (see *gambiae* complex above). More or less permanent waters, especially with vegetation, such as swamps, marshes, edges of streams, rivers and ditches. Prefers shaded habitats. Bites man predominantly, but also domestic animals, feeds indoors and also outdoors, after feeding rests mainly indoors, but also outdoors.

Other *Anopheles*
An. nili, *An. moucheti*, *An. hargreavesi* and *An. pharoensis* may also be malaria vectors of minor importance in certain localities.

Malaria vectors of North Africa and the Middle East

(Morocco, Libya, Egypt, Turkey, Syria, Iran, Iraq and Saudi
Arabia, etc.)

An. atroparvus
England across Europe to the Caspian Sea and southwards to
Spain. Formerly an important European vector but now transmits
malaria in only a few areas. Larvae occur in sunlit, exposed pools
and ditches with either fresh or brackish water, they also breed
in rice fields. Adults bite man and also domestic animals. Commonly found in stables, cow sheds and piggeries. During the
winter females enter partial hibernation, sheltering in houses or
animal quarters, periodically emerging to bite people or livestock.

An. claviger
England through Europe to North Africa, Israel, Iran, Iraq and
Asia Minor to Afghanistan, but vector only in Middle East and
Mediterranean countries. Ponds, marshes, wells, cisterns and rock
pools, sunlight or shade. Bites man and domestic animals indoors
and outdoors, and after feeding rests indoors or outdoors.

An. labranchiae
England through Europe to Morocco, Algeria and Tunisia, now
a vector only in North Africa. Brackish waters in coastal marshes,
fresh waters of rice fields, marshes and edges of grassy streams
and ditches, prefers sunlight. Bites man and also domestic animals
indoors and outdoors, rests mainly in houses or animal shelters
after feeding.

An. pharoensis
Israel, Saudi Arabia, Syria, Egypt and most of Africa south of the
Sahara, only a vector of importance in Egypt. Marshes, swamps,
rice fields and ponds, especially those with abundant grassy or
floating vegetation. Bites man and animals, indoors or outdoors,
rests outdoors after feeding.

An. sacharovi
Italy, Greece, Eastern Europe, Israel, Turkey, Syria, Jordan,
Lebanon, Iran, Iraq to Central Russia; malaria vector in
Israel and Middle East countries. Fresh or brackish waters of

coastal or inland marshes, pools, ponds, especially those with vegetation. Prefers sunlit habitats. Bites man and animals indoors or outdoors, usually rests in houses or animal shelters after feeding.

An. sergentii

Canary Islands, Algeria, Tunisia, Egypt, Syria, Israel, Turkey, Afghanistan and Pakistan to north-west India; vector in Egypt, Israel and Saudi Arabia. Rice fields, borrow pits, ditches, seepages, slow flowing streams, sunlit or partially shaded habitats. Bites man or animals indoors or outdoors, rests in houses and caves after feeding.

An. stephensi (includes mysorensis)

Egypt, Iraq, Iran, Saudi Arabia, Oman, Dubai, Bahrain, Afghanistan, Pakistan, Sri Lanka, India, Burma, Thailand and China. An important vector over much of its range, especially in and around towns. Breeds in man-made habitats associated with towns, such as cisterns, wells, gutters, water-storage jars and containers, drains, fresh or brackish waters, and even polluted waters, and in rural situations in grassy pools and alongside rivers. Adults bite man indoors and outdoors and rest mainly indoors after feeding.

An. superpictus

Greece, Mediterranean area, Iran, Iraq, Saudi Arabia, Israel, Jordan, Turkey, Afghanistan and Pakistan. Flowing waters such as torrents of shallow water over rocky streams, pools in rivers, muddy hill streams, vegetation may be present, prefers sunlight. Bites man and animals indoors and outdoors, after feeding rests mainly in houses and animal shelters, also in caves.

Malaria vectors of the Indian Subcontinent

(Afghanistan, Pakistan, India, Nepal, Bengal, Sri Lanka, Bangladesh, etc.).

An. culicifacies

Oman, Bahrain, Afghanistan, Pakistan through India, Sri Lanka, Bangladesh, Burma, Thailand, Indochina and southern China; probably most important vector in much of Pakistan, India, Bangladesh and Sri Lanka. Great variety of clean and polluted habitats, irrigation ditches, rice fields, swamps, pools, wells, borrow pits, edges of streams and occasionally in brackish waters. Sunlit or partially shaded habitats. Prefers domestic animals but commonly bites man indoors or outdoors, rests mainly indoors after feeding.

An. fluviatilis
Oman, Bahrain, Iran, Iraq, eastern Saudi Arabia, Pakistan, Afghanistan, India, Sri Lanka, Bangladesh, Burma, Thailand, Indonesia, Indochina, China and Taiwan. Important vector in Pakistan, India and Bangladesh. Most flowing waters, such as hill streams, pools in river beds, irrigation ditches, prefers sunlight. Bites man and also domestic animals indoors and outdoors, rests both indoors and outdoors after feeding.

An. minimus (includes flavirostris)
India, Sri Lanka, Burma, Malaysia, Thailand, Indochina, Taiwan, Sumatra, Java, and the Philippines to southern China. Flowing waters, such as foothill streams, springs, irrigation ditches, seepages, also rice fields and borrow pits. Prefers shaded areas of sunlit habitats. Feeds mainly on man, but also domestic animals, also feeds and rests mainly indoors. In the Philippines the subspecies *flavirostris* bites indoors but rests outdoors after feeding. Some authorities regard *flavirostris* as a distinct species, not a subspecies of *An. minimus*.

An. stephensi
See North Africa and Middle East.

An. sundaicus
India, Burma, Malaysia, Thailand, Indonesia, Java, Sumatra, Borneo, Taiwan, China and Indochina. Salt or brackish waters, lagoons, marshes, pools and seepages, especially with putrifying algae and aquatic weeds, mainly a coastal species, but found in freshwater inland pools in Java and Sumatra. Prefers sunlight. Bites man and domestic animals indoors and outdoors, and rests mainly indoors after feeding.

An. superpictus
See North Africa and Middle East.

An. varuna

India, Sri Lanka, Bangladesh, Nepal, Burma and Thailand, This species is similar to *An. minimus* and has often been confused with it. It appears to be a malaria vector in central and northern India. Larvae occur in stagnant ditches, pools, slow-running streams, wells in sunlit or shaded conditions. Bites man and animals indoors and outdoors, commonly rests indoors after feeding. Vector mainly in hilly and forested areas of east-central India.

Malaria vectors in South-east Asia

(Assam, Burma, Thailand, Indochina, Indonesia, Malaysia, Philippines, etc).

An. aconitus

Eastern India, Sri Lanka, Malaysia, Indochina, Indonesia and southern China. Rice fields, swamps, irrigation ditches, pools and streams with vegetation, prefers sunlit habitats. Adults feed indoors or outdoors on man but also commonly on animals, adults rest indoors or outdoors after feeding.

An. campestris

There has been considerable confusion over the identity of this species, it has sometimes been misidentified as *An. donaldi* but more frequently as *An. barbirostris*. Many references in the literature refer to *An. barbirostris* as an important vector of both malaria and filariasis, but it is predominantly zoophagic and the real vector is *An. campestris*. Consequently most references giving *An. barbirostris* as a vector refer, in fact, to *An. campestris*, a species found along the coasts and deltas of Malaysia and Thailand and possibly in other mainland areas of South-east Asia. Larvae in deep waters usually having some vegetation. Partial shade is preferred, larvae often accumulate in shaded corners of rice fields, also ditches, earthen wells and sometimes in brackish waters. Bites man and animals indoors and outdoors, substantial numbers rest indoors after feeding.

An culicifacies

See Indian subcontinent.

An. hyrcanus

This mosquito has been reported from Europe, the northern Mediterranean, North Africa, across central and northern Asia to Japan, but what was formerly considered a single species is now known to consist of a species group. Many records incriminating *An. hyrcanus* in the transmission of malaria refer to closely related species such as *An. lesteri*, *An. sinensis* and *An. nigerrimus*. In these brief notes these species have been identified as malaria vectors, but not *An. hyrcanus* sensu stricto, although it may be a vector in some areas.

An. lesteri and An. sinensis of hyrcanus group

There has been much taxonomic confusion over the different mosquitoes in this group, some forms occur in northern Mediterranean areas, others in India, and several in the Far East. *An. sinensis* was considered an important vector in China, but this was probably partly based on misidentification. The most important vector in the group is probably *An. lesteri*. This species occurs in Thailand, Malaysia, Borneo, Philippines, Korea and southern China to Japan. Larvae in cool, clean waters, some forms can occur in brackish water, prefers shaded habitats. Bites man and animals indoors and outdoors, rests indoors and outdoors after feeding.

An. letifer and An. umbrosus

India, Thailand, Indonesia, Malaysia, Philippines, Sumatra and Borneo. *An. letifer* is very similar to *An. umbrosus* which has a similar distribution and has, in the past, been confused with it. *An. umbrosus*, however, is probably not such an important malaria vector as formerly supposed, many sporozoites found in its salivary glands are probably of rodent malarias. *An. letifer* bites man more often than *An. umbrosus*, but also commonly feeds on animals, and seems to be a malaria vector in certain areas. Larvae often live in stagnant waters, such as pools, swamps and ponds, especially on coastal plains, prefer shade. Bites animals and man mainly outdoors, rests outdoors after feeding.

An. leucosphyrus group

There is still confusion concerning the identity of three very similar species within this group, namely *An. leucosphyrus*, *An. balabacensis* and *An. dirus*. *An. leucosphyrus* occurs in Indonesia,

Sumatra, Malaysia, Sabah and Sarawak. Larvae commonly occur in clear seepage pools in forests. Adults bite man inside or outside houses, but afterwards rest outdoors. It is a vector in Sumatra and Sarawak and possibly elsewhere. *An. balabacensis* occurs from western India through Burma, Thailand, Vietnam, northern Malaysia, Sabah, Philippines and southern China. It is also a forest species. Larvae colonise muddy and shaded forest pools, animal hoof prints and vehicle ruts. Adults bite man and cattle. Feed and rest outdoors. In Thailand and possibly elsewhere, *An. dirus* a species very similar both morphologically and biologically to *An. balabacensis*, is an important malaria vector.

An. maculatus
India, Sri Lanka, Malaysia, Indonesia, Indochina, Borneo, Taiwan, Philippines and southern China. Found in or near hilly areas, in seepage waters, pools formed in streams, edges of ponds, ditches and swamps with much vegetation, prefers sunlight. Bites man and animals mainly outdoors and rests mainly outdoors after feeding.

An. minimus
See Indian subcontinent.

An. nigerrimus
Formerly regarded as a subspecies of *An. hyrcanus*. India, Sri Lanka, Burma, Thailand, Malaysia, Indochina, Borneo and China. Larvae in deep ponds, rice fields, irrigation ditches and swamps with much vegetation, prefers sunlight. Bites man and animals mainly outdoors and rests mainly outdoors after feeding.

An. subpictus
Iran, Pakistan, India, Sri Lanka, Burma, Malaysia, Thailand, Indonesia, Indochina, China, New Guinea, Java and Celebes. May be important malaria vector in Celebes, Java and Indochina. Larvae in muddy pools near houses, gutters, borrow pits, also in brackish waters. Bites mainly animals but also man both indoors and outdoors, rests indoors or outdoors after feeding.

An. sundaicus
See Indian subcontinent.

Malaria vectors of China, Taiwan and Korea

An. balabacensis
Important vector in jungle areas of Hainan. See South-east Asia.

An. lesteri
Principal vector in central plains of China. Larvae in cool clean waters, they prefer shade. Adults bite man and animals outdoors, rest indoors and outdoors.

An. pattoni
China, north of about the 30th parallel. Larvae in pools in or near streams, and rock pools, especially in habitats with algae, prefers sunlight. Bites man indoors and outdoors.

An. sinensis
Probably not so important as formerly believed, but a vector in central and southern areas of China. Larvae in swamps, rice fields and grassy ponds. Adults bite man and cattle outdoors, and rest outdoors.

Malaria vectors of the Australasian area

An. bancroftii
New Guinea, Australia and Bismarck Archipelago. Larvae in permanent waters, usually with vegetation, shaded or sunlit. Adults bite man and animals outdoors, and rest outdoors after feeding.

An. punctulatus complex
Moluccas, New Guinea, Solomon Islands, New Hebrides to northern Australia. This is a species complex consisting of at least four species; *An. punctulatus*, *An. farauti* spp. 'No. 1' and 'No. 2', and *An. koliensis*. All four species are malaria vectors. In general larval habitats are swamps, edges of slow flowing streams, springs, puddles, hoof prints, pools, wells, water-storage containers and other man-made receptacles. Water may be either fresh, slightly brackish or even polluted and in sunlight or shade. Adults bite man indoors or outdoors and rest indoors or outdoors after feeding, but in New Guinea rest mainly outdoors. *An. koliensis* seems to prefer to breed in marshy pools or pools at edges of

forest streams. Adults usually bite man and rest after feeding outdoors.

Filariasis (see Table 3.1)

Certain *Anopheles* species transmit filarial worms of *Wuchereria bancrofti*, *Brugia malayi*, and *Brugia timori*, all of which cause filariasis in man.

W. bancrofti causes filariasis in people living in most tropical regions of the world (Central and South America, Africa and Asia, including the Pacific area), and also in some subtropical areas such as the Mediterranean region and Australia. In many of these areas bancroftian filariasis is mainly an urban disease. In contrast *B. malayi* is more of a rural disease and has a more restricted distribution occurring only in Asia, in countries such as southern India, Malaysia, Indonesia, Thailand, Indochina, China, New Guinea, Philippines and Polynesia. Both diseases occur in two basic forms: nocturnal periodic and nocturnal subperiodic (sometimes called aperiodic).

In the nocturnal periodic forms of these two parasites, most of the microfilariae in man are in the blood vessels supplying the internal organs, such as the lungs, during the day. At night, however, especially during the middle part, they migrate to the peripheral blood system and lymph vessels. Because of this marked diel (24 h) periodicity microfilariae are mainly ingested by mosquitoes feeding on man at night. *Anopheles* mosquitoes which bite man mainly at night are therefore among the vectors of the nocturnal periodic form of *W. bancrofti*, which is found throughout most of the tropics except in the Pacific (where it is replaced by the diurnal subperiodic form). *Anopheles* are also vectors of the periodic form of *B. malayi* which is found more or less throughout the range of the parasite.

The mosquitoes involved in filareasis transmission differ according to the area, but many of the principal malaria vectors are also important filarial vectors. For example, *An. nigerrimus*, *An. aconitus*, *An. flavirostris*, *An. philippinensis*, *An. darlingi*, *An. punctulatus* complex, *An. letifer*, *An. funestus*, *An. gambiae* complex, *An. aquasalis*, *An. sinensis*, *An. minimus*, *An. maculatus*, etc., are all vectors of nocturnal periodic *W. bancrofti*; while *An. barbirostris*, *An. campestris*, *An. sinensis* and others are vectors of the nocturnal periodic form of *B. malayi*. Female *Anopheles* can be infected with both malarial and filarial parasites and thus transmit both diseases. (Other night-biting mosquitoes such as *Culex* and *Mansonia* species are also vectors of nocturnal periodic and subperiodic filariasis—see Table 3.1).

In subperiodic *W. bancrofti* and *B. malayi* the microfilariae exhibit a reduced periodicity and are present in the peripheral blood during the day as well as at night, but there remains some degree of periodicity. For example, subperiodic *W. bancrofti* (which is found in Polynesia) has a small peak in microfilarial density during the daytime and can therefore be called diurnally subperiodic, whereas subperiodic *B. malayi* in West Malaysia, South Vietnam, Thailand, Sabah, and the Palewan Islands exhibits a slight peak of microfilariae at night and can be called nocturnally subperiodic. (Culicine mosquitoes which bite during the daytime, such as certain *Mansonia* and *Aedes* species, are important vectors of subperiodic filariasis—see Table 3.1).

Filarial development of *W. bancrofti* and *B. malayi* within the mosquito vector, and the basic mode of transmission from mosquito to man is the same for all vectors. Basically, the life-cycle in the mosquito is as follows. Microfilariae ingested with the blood-meal pass into the stomach of the mosquito (in some vectors such as *Anopheles* many may be destroyed during their passage through the oesophagus). Within a few minutes they exsheath, penetrate the stomach wall and pass into the haemocele, from where they migrate to the thoracic muscles of the mosquito. In the thorax the small larvae become more or less inactive, grow shorter but considerably fatter and develop, after 2 days, into 'sausage-shaped' forms. They undergo two moults and the resultant 3rd-stage larvae become active, leave the muscles and migrate through the head and down the fleshy labium of the proboscis. This is the infective stage and is formed some 10 days or more after the microfilariae have been ingested with a blood-meal.

When the mosquito takes further blood-meals, infective (3rd-stage) larvae (about 1.2–1.6 mm long) rupture the skin of the labella of the labium and crawl onto the surface of the host's skin. Several infective larvae may be liberated onto the skin when a vector is biting. However, many of these small worms die. Only a few manage to find a skin abrasion, sometimes the small lesion caused by the mosquito's bite, and thus enter the skin and pass to the lymphatic system. It should be noted that the salivary glands are not involved in the transmission of filariasis, and also that there is no multiplication or sexual cycle of the parasites in the mosquito.

There are no known animal reservoirs of *W. bancrofti*; it is a disease solely of man.

In contrast *Brugia malayi* is a zoonosis. The nocturnal subperiodic form is essentially a parasite of swamp-inhabiting monkeys, especially the so-called 'leaf monkeys' (*Presbytis* spp.); man becomes infected when he lives at the edges of these areas. Other reservoirs include wild and domestic cats, dogs and pangolins. The nocturnal periodic form is more adapted to man and there do not appear to be any important animal reservoirs, but in some areas monkeys may act as reservoirs.

Infection rates of infective larvae in anopheline vectors vary according to the mosquito species and local conditions, but they are often about 0.1–5 per cent for *W. bancrofti* and from about 0.1–3 per cent for *Brugia malayi*.

Brugia timori is known only from Timor island in Indonesia. Its microfilariae are nocturnally periodic and are transmitted to man by *Anopheles* mosquitoes such as *An. barbirostris*.

The presence of filarial worms in the thoracic muscles of mosquitoes, or infective worms in the proboscis, does not necessarily implicate mosquitoes as vectors of bancroftian or brugian filariasis. This is because there are several other mosquito-transmitted filariae. For example, various *Setaria* species infecting cattle, *Dirofilaria repens* and *Dirofilaria immitis* infecting dogs, and various other species of *Brugia*, such as *B. patei* in Africa and *B. pahangi* in Asia infect animals but not man. Careful examination is therefore essential to identify the filarial parasites found in mosquitoes as those of *W. bancrofti* or *Brugia malayi*.

Table 3.1 (p. 81) summarises the distribution and vectors of filariasis.

Arboviruses

The word arboviruses is derived from the term '*arthropod-borne-virus*'. An arbovirus infection in either man or non-human hosts produces viraemia; the virus is ingested by blood-sucking insects such as mosquitoes when they take blood-meals. Within the vector the virus undergoes multiplication and/or cyclical development before being transmitted by the infected arthropod during refeeding. An arbovirus therefore undergoes obligatory development in an arthropod host; yellow fever and dengue are typical arboviruses transmitted by *Aedes* mosquitoes. In contrast the virus causing poliomyelitis is not an arbovirus for although it can be transmitted by certain flies, such as houseflies, this is purely mechanical transmission; the virus does not undergo any multiplication and/or development in an arthropod. The time taken for the infected mosquito to become infective, that is the extrinsic incubation period of the arbovirus, varies according to temperature, the species of arbovirus and mosquito. There are known to be at least 109 different arboviruses, but, taking into consideration about another 73 viruses probably transmitted by arthropods and about 238 that are also possibly arboviruses, the total is about 420. Many arboviruses are transmitted by culicine mosquitoes, in particular *Aedes* and *Culex* species, others are spread by ticks and other arthropods.

In 1959–60 a major epidemic of a painful but non-fatal disease, called O'nyong nyong (an African word meaning 'joint-breaker') was identified in Uganda and Kenya, and later in other countries of East and Central Africa. It was discovered that it was spread by the *An. gambiae* complex and *An. funestus*. This was the first time an *Anopheles* mosquito was incriminated with the spread of any arbovirus. About 20 other arboviruses of man have since been found to be transmitted by *Anopheles*, some are also transmitted by culicine mosquitoes but others are known only, or principally, from *Anopheles*. Examples are Guaroa (*An. neivai*: man, Colombia), Nyando and Tanga (*An. funestus*: man, East Africa), Tataguine (*An. funestus* and *An. gambiae* complex: man, West Africa) and Kowanyama and Trubanaman (*An. annulipes*: man, fowl, horses, kangaroos, Australia).

CONTROL

The principal methods of mosquito control are outlined in the preceding chapter. Here only methods specifically directed at *Anopheles* are considered.

In certain areas predatory fish such as *Gambusia* have reduced larval populations but it is debatable whether this has ever led to any significant reduction in disease transmission. Paris green dusts and larvicidal oils were used extensively prior to the introduction of the residual insecticides. When used consistently they helped reduce malaria transmission in localised areas of economic or social importance, such as principal towns, coffee and tea estates, rubber plantations and mining encampments.

Draining swamps and marshes has in some areas reduced the numbers of *Anopheles* vectors, but draining, or filling-in habitats, is impracticable against some important vectors. For example, larvae of the *An. gambiae* complex, principal malaria vectors in Africa, occur in temporary small pools and puddles while those of *An. balabacensis*, an important vector in South-east Asia, occur in forest swamps. In both these situations water management control procedures are not feasible.

Residual house-spraying

In most malaria campaigns control is now focused on the adults. The most widely practised method is the application of water dispersable powders of residual insecticides to the interior surface of walls, ceilings and roofs of houses. In the absence of resistance DDT is the best insecticide, and this is usually sprayed as a water dispersable (wettable) powder at the rate of $2\,\mathrm{g\,m}^{-2}$. Even in highly endemic areas houses need be sprayed only at 6 monthly intervals, and where malaria transmission is very seasonal a single spraying a year may be sufficient to give good control.

Alternative organochlorine insecticides are HCH, which is normally applied at a recommended dose of $0.4\,\mathrm{g\,m}^{-2}$ three-to-four times a year, and dieldrin at the rate of $0.6\,\mathrm{g\,m}^{-2}$, once a year. Dieldrin and HCH are more toxic to mosquitoes, and man, than DDT, and HCH is more volatile than either DDT or dieldrin. The safest of these three insecticides is DDT, dieldrin is the most toxic and should only be used for indoor spraying under strict safety measures. One of the few disadvantages of DDT is that it may be an irritant to mosquitoes, causing them to leave sprayed surfaces before they have picked up a lethal dose.

If mosquitoes are resistant to DDT then organophosphate insecticides such as malathion, fenthion (Baytex), fenitrothion (Sumithion), or carbamates such as carbaryl (Sevin) and propoxur (Baygon) can be used, at rates of about $1.5\text{–}2.0\,\mathrm{g\,m}^{-2}$. However, these organophosphate and carbamate insecticides are less persistent, and spraying may have to be repeated at 3–4 monthly intervals. They are also many times more expensive than DDT and the increased number of spraying cycles needed will again increase costs. Furthermore, they are more toxic to man than DDT and greater safety measures have to be introduced during control campaigns.

The effectiveness of residual spraying of houses depends on the indoor resting habits of the mosquitoes. It is not essential, however, that malaria vectors are killed on the first contact with sprayed surfaces because *Anopheles* must live at least 10–14 days before they can transmit malaria. Therefore, even if they need several periods of contact with insecticides before they are killed, malaria transmission will still be prevented, that is so long as their longevity is reduced to less than 10–14 days. It is possible, therefore, to have large biting populations of vectors too young to transmit malaria. In practice, however, anophelines are usually killed by residual insecticides at an early age. This results in a decrease in numbers of ovipositions and eventually large reductions in the population size of vectors. If, however, spraying ceases, any remaining small populations of vectors can build up again, and if malarial parasites are still present in the human population a recrudescence of malaria transmission is likely to follow. Even if malaria vectors have been completely eradicated by insecticidal spraying, there remains the possibility that the area will be reinvaded by mosquitoes flying in from outside, and breeding become re-established.

Alternative control measures

It has become increasingly obvious that many malaria vectors, especially some of those in Central and South America and South-east Asia, are unfortunately exophilic, hence spraying houses with residual insecticides will be of little use in reducing malaria. Another problem with house spraying is that it may alter the behaviour of the vector population. For example, house spraying may kill the endophilic proportion of the vector population, but by so doing reduce competition between the larvae of endophilic and exophilic adults which occur in the same breeding places. This could allow an increase in the production of exophilic adults. Consequently, after some years of house spraying there may be a substantial increase in the exophilic, and possibly exophagic, proportion of the vector population, with the result that malaria again becomes a problem because of large outdoor resting and biting populations. Alternative control measures are needed to combat these difficulties. One method is to use outdoor aerosol applications of malathion, synthetic pyrethroids or some other suitable insecticide. In addition to killing the exophilic populations this method may also kill the indoor resting adults if the insecticidal fog penetrates houses. Mosquito nets and mosquito screening can reduce the risk of acquiring malaria and other mosquito-borne diseases, but such measures will not be effective against vectors that bite during the day or early evening, that is, before people have gone to bed. Another approach is to focus attention on larvicides.

It seems unlikely that efficient malaria control will be achieved or maintained, by relying on a single method of attack. Malaria is most likely to be conquered by integrated control, incorporating improvements in housing, general hygiene and education. Even so, it seems that it will be a long time before the complex problem of malaria is solved.

Malaria contro and malaria eradication

In 1955 the eighth World Health Assembly stated that worldwide malaria eradication, except in Africa south of the Sahara, was technically feasible. However, a sense of urgency in achieving this aim was recognised because insecticide resistance in *Anopheles* had been reported in 1950. In 1968 the 22nd World Health Assembly realised it had been over optimistic and declared that global malaria eradication was not at present possible although it remained the ultimate goal, and that for the time being malaria control should be the aim. This is still the strategy today: that is control whenever feasible.

The difference between malaria eradication and malaria control is that malaria eradication means the total cessation of transmission and elimination of the reservoir of infection in man so that at the end of the anti-malaria campaign there is no resumption of transmission. Malaria control means reducing malaria transmission to an acceptable rate, that is to a level that no longer constitutes a major public health problem. This has the implication that control measures have to be maintained indefinitely; if they are relaxed malaria prevalence will rise. The feasibility of control will depend, not only on scientific considerations, but also on the financial and public health resources of the community, or country.

Chapter 3
Culicine Mosquitoes

The subfamily Culicinae contains 33 genera of mosquitoes, of which the medically most important ones are *Culex*, *Aedes*, *Mansonia*, *Sabethes* and *Haemagogus*. The genera *Culex*, *Aedes* and *Mansonia* are found in both temperate regions and throughout all tropical areas, but *Haemagogus* and *Sabethes* are found in only Central and South America.

Certain *Aedes* mosquitoes are vectors of yellow fever in Africa, while *Aedes*, *Haemogogus* and *Sabethes* are yellow fever vectors in Central and South America. *Aedes* species are also vectors of the classical and haemorrhagic forms of dengue. All five genera of culicine mosquitoes mentioned here, as well as some others, can transmit a variety of other arboviruses. Some *Culex*, *Aedes* and *Mansonia* species are important vectors of filariasis (*Wuchereria bancrofti* or *Brugia malayi*).

Characters separating the subfamily Culicinae from the Anophelinae have been given in Chapter 1 and are summarised in Table 1.1.

It is not easy to give a reliable and non-technical guide to the identification of the five most important culicine genera. Nevertheless, characters that will usually separate these genera are given below, together with notes on their biology. Only people working in Central and South America need to recognise *Haemagogus* and *Sabethes* mosquitoes.

CULEX MOSQUITOES

Distribution

More or less world-wide, but they are absent from the extreme northern parts of the temperate zones.

Eggs

Usually brown, long and cylindrical, laid upright on the water surface and placed together to form an egg raft which can comprise up to about 300 eggs (see Fig. 1.15). No glue or cement-like substance binds the eggs to each other; adhesion is due to surface forces holding the eggs together. Eggs of a few other mosquitoes, including those of the subgenus *Coquillettidia* of *Mansonia*, also deposit their eggs in rafts.

Larvae

The siphon is often long and narrow (Fig. 3.1), but it may be short and fat. There is always more than one pair of subventral tufts of hairs on the siphon, none of which is near its base. These hair tufts may consist of very few short and simple hairs which may be missed unless larvae are carefully examined under a microscope.

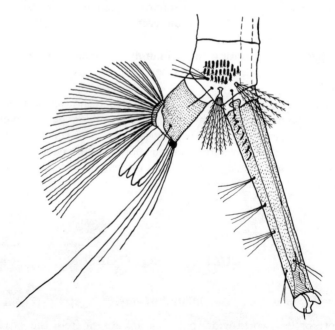

Fig. 3.1 Terminal segment of a *Culex* larva showing long siphon with three subventral tufts of hairs.

Adults

Frequently, but not always, the thorax, legs and wing veins are covered with sombre coloured, often brown, scales. The abdomen is often covered with brown or blackish scales but some whitish scales may occur on most segments. Adults are recognised more by their lack of ornamentation than any striking diagnostic characters. The tip of the abdomen of females is blunt. The claws of all tarsi are simple and those of the hind tarsi are very small. Examination under a microscope shows that all tarsi have a pair of small fleshy pulvilli (see Fig. 1.2).

Biology

Eggs are laid in a great variety of aquatic habitats. Most *Culex* species breed in ground collections of water such as pools, puddles, ditches, borrow pits and rice fields. Some lay eggs in manmade container habitats such as tin cans, water receptables, bottles and storage tanks. Only a few species breed in tree holes and even fewer in leaf axils. The most important species, *Culex quinquefasciatus* which is a filariasis vector, breeds in waters polluted with organic debris such as rotting vegetation, household refuse and excreta. Larvae of this vector species are commonly found in partially blocked drains and ditches, soak-away pits, septic tanks and in village pots, especially the abandoned ones in which water is polluted and unfit for drinking. It is a mosquito that is associated with urbanisation, and towns with poor and inadequate drainage and sanitation. Under these conditions its population increases rapidly.

Culex tritaeniorhynchus is an important vector of Japanese encephalitis and breeds prolifically in cleaner habitats especially rice fields. In southern Asia larvae are not uncommon in slightly polluted waters such as fish ponds which have had manure added.

Culex quinquefasciatus, and many other *Culex* species, bite man and other hosts at night. Some species, like *Cx. quinquefasciatus*, commonly rest indoors both before and after feeding, but they also shelter in outdoor resting places.

AEDES MOSQUITOES

Distribution

World-wide, their range extends well into northern and Arctic areas where they can be vicious biters and serious pests to man and livestock.

Eggs

Eggs are usually black, more or less ovoid in shape and are always laid singly (see Fig. 1.15). Careful examination shows that the egg shell has a distinctive mosaic pattern. Eggs are laid on damp substrates just beyond the water line, such as on damp mud and leaf litter of pools, on the damp walls of clay pots, rock pools and tree holes.

Aedes eggs can withstand desiccation, the intensity and duration of which varies, but in many species they can remain dry, but viable, for many months. When flooded, some eggs may hatch within a few minutes, others of the same batch may require prolonged immersion in water, thus hatching may be spread over several days or weeks. Even when eggs are soaked for long periods some may fail to hatch because they require several soakings followed by short periods of desiccation before hatching can be induced. Even if environmental conditions are favourable, eggs may be in a state of diapause and will not hatch until this resting period is terminated. Various stimuli including reduction in the oxygen content of water, changes in daylength, and temperature may be required to break diapause in *Aedes* eggs.

Many *Aedes* species breed in small container habitats (tree holes, plant axils, etc.) which are susceptible to drying out, thus the ability of eggs to withstand desiccation is clearly advantageous. Desiccation and the ability of *Aedes* eggs to hatch in instalments can create problems with controlling the immature stages (p. 84).

Larvae

Aedes species have a short barrel-shaped siphon and only one pair of subventral tufts (Fig. 3.2) which never arises less than one-quarter of the distance from the base of the siphon. Additional characters are at least three pairs of setae in the ventral brush, the

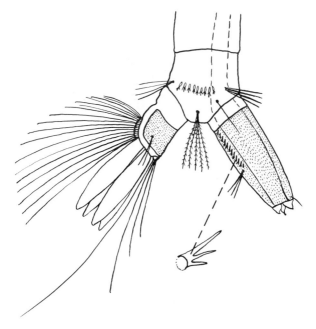

Fig. 3.2 Terminal segments of an *Aedes* larva showing short siphon with a single subventral tuft.

antennae are not greatly flattened and there are no enormous setae on the thorax. These characters should separate *Aedes* larvae from most of the culicine genera, but not unfortunately from larvae of South American *Haemagogus*. In Central and South America *Aedes* larvae can usually be distinguished from those of *Haemagogus*, by possession of either larger or more strongly spiculate antennae; also the comb is not on a sclerotised plate as in some *Haemagogus*.

Adults

Many, but not all, *Aedes* adults have conspicuous patterns on the thorax formed by black, white or silvery scales (Fig. 3.3a); in some species yellow scales are present. The legs often have black and white rings (Fig. 3.4b). *Aedes aegypti*, often called the yellow fever mosquito, is readily recognised by the 'lyre'-shaped silver markings on the lateral edges of the scutum (Fig. 3.3a). Scales on the wing veins of *Aedes* mosquitoes are narrow, and are usually

Chapter 3

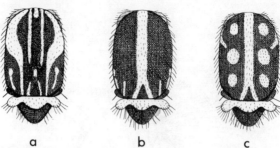

a   b   c

Fig. 3.3 Dorsal surface of the thoraces of adult *Aedes* mosquitoes showing pattern of black and white scales. (a) *Aedes aegypti* with typical 'lyre'-shaped markings; (b) *Ae. albopictus;* (c) *Ae. vittatus.*

more or less all black, except may be at the base of the wing. In *Aedes* the abdomen is often covered with black and white scales forming distinctive patterns, and in the female it is pointed at the tip (Fig. 3.4a).

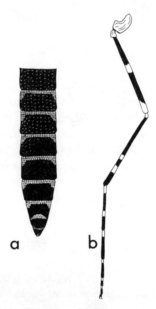

a   b

Fig. 3.4 *Aedes* adults showing arrangement of black and white scales. (a) Abdomen; (b) leg.

Biology

Although some *Aedes* species breed in ground pools, many, especially tropical species, are found in natural or man-made container habitats such as tree holes, bamboo stumps, leaf axils, rock pools, village pots, tin cans and tyres. For example, *Ae. aegypti* breeds in village pots and water-storage jars placed either inside or outside houses. Larvae occur mainly in those with clean water intended for drinking. In some areas *Ae. aegypti* also breeds in rock pools and tree holes. *Aedes africanas*, an African species involved in the sylvatic transmission of yellow fever, breeds mainly in tree holes and bamboo stumps, whereas *Ae. simpsoni*, another African yellow-fever vector, breeds almost exclusively in leaf axils, especially those of banana plants, yams and pineapples. *Aedes albopictus*, vector of dengue in South-east Asia, resembles *Ae. aegypti* in breeding principally in domestic containers. Larvae of *Ae. polynesiensis* occur in man-made and natural containers, especially split coconut shells, and larvae of *Ae. pseudoscutellaris* are found mainly in tree holes and bamboo stumps. Both of these last two mosquitoes are important vectors of diurnal subperiodic bancroftian filariasis. *Aedes togoi*, a vector of bancroftian and brugian filariasis, breeds principally in rock pools containing fresh or brackish water.

The life-cycle from egg to adult can take as little as 6-7 days, but it is often 10-12 days and much longer in temperate climates.

Adults of most *Aedes* species bite mainly during the day or early evening. Most biting occurs outdoors and adults usually rest out of doors although larval habitats may be water-storage jars placed inside houses.

HAEMAGOGUS MOSQUITOES

Distribution

Found only in Central and South America.

Eggs

Usually black and ovoid and laid singly in tree holes and other natural container habitats, occasionally in man-made ones. There is no simple method of distinguishing *Haemagogus* eggs from those of *Aedes* mosquitoes.

Larvae

Larvae have a single subventral tuft arising, as in *Aedes* larvae, not less than a quarter of the distance from the base of the siphon. They resemble *Aedes* larvae but can usually be separated by the following combination of characters: antennae short and either without, or with only very few, spicules, a ventral brush arising from a sclerotised boss (Fig. 3.5). In some species the comb teeth are at the edge of a sclerotised plate, in *Aedes* this plate is absent.

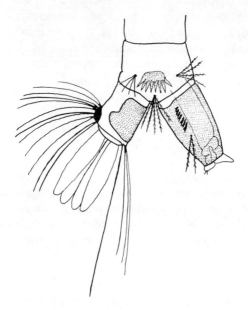

Fig. 3.5 Terminal segments of *Haemagogus* larva showing ventral brush arising from a dark sclerotised boss, and comb scales arranged on a small plate.

Adults

Adults are very colourful and they can easily be recognised by the presence of broad, flat and bright metallic blue, red, green or golden coloured scales, covering the dorsal part of the thorax.

Like *Sabethes* mosquitoes they have exceptionally large anterior pronotal thoracic lobes (see Fig. 3.7) behind the head. *Haemagogus* adults are rather similar to *Sabethes* in other respects, and it may be difficult for the novice to separate these two genera. However, no *Haemagogus* mosquito has paddles on the legs, which is a conspicuous feature of many, but not all, species of *Sabethes*.

Biology

Egg can withstand desiccation. Larvae occur mostly in tree holes and bamboo stumps, but also in rock pools, split coconut shells and sometimes in assorted domestic containers. They are basically forest mosquitoes. Adults bite during the day, but mostly in the tree tops where they feed on monkeys. Under certain environmental conditions, however, such as experienced at edges of forests, during tree felling operations or during the dry season, they may descend to the forest floor to bite man and other hosts. *Haemagogus spegazzinii*, *Hg. equinus*, *Hg. leucocelaenus* (this species was previously placed in the genus *Aedes*), *Hg. jathinomys* (=*falco*) and *Hg. capricornii* are all involved in yellow fever transmission in forest areas.

SABETHES MOSQUITOES

Distribution

Found only in Central and South America.

Eggs

Little is known about the eggs of *Sabethes* species, but it appears that they are laid singly, have no prominent surface features such as bosses or sculpturing and are incapable of withstanding desiccation. The eggs of *Sabethes chloropterus*, a species sometimes involved in the sylvatic cycle of yellow fever, are rhomboid in shape and can thus be readily identified from most other culicine eggs (see Fig. 3.7b).

Larvae

The siphon has many hairs placed ventrally, laterally or dorsally, and is relatively slender and moderately long (Fig. 3.6). *Sabethes* larvae can usually be distinguished from other mosquito larvae by having only one pair of setae in the ventral brush, the comb teeth arranged in a single row, or at most with 3–4 detached teeth, and by the absence of a pecten.

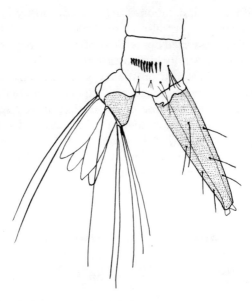

Fig. 3.6 Terminal segments of a *Sabethes* larva showing single pair of hairs in ventral brush, numerous simple hairs on the siphon, and absence on siphon of a pecten.

Adults

The dorsal surface of the thorax is covered with appressed iridescent blue, green and red scales. The anterior pronotal lobes are very large (Fig. 3.7a). Adults of many species have one or more pairs of tarsi with conspicuous paddles composed of narrow scales. Their presence immediately distinguishes *Sabethes* from all other mosquitoes (Fig. 3.7c). Species which lack these paddles resemble those of *Haemagogus* and a specialist is required to identify them.

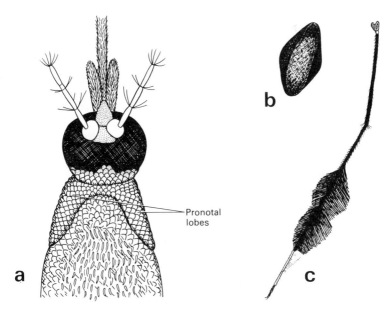

Fig. 3.7 *Sabethes* mosquitoes. (a) Head and thorax showing pronotal lobes forming a 'collar' behind the head; (b) an egg; (c) hind leg showing narrow scales forming a paddle.

Biology

Larvae occur in tree holes and bamboo stumps; a few species are found in leaf axils of bromeliads and other plants. They are forest mosquitoes. They bite during the day, mainly in the tree canopy, but like *Haemagogus* adults, may descend to ground le el at certain times to bite man and other hosts. *Sabethes chloropterus* has been incriminated as a sylvan vector of yellow fever.

MANSONIA MOSQUITOES

Distribution

Principally a genus of wet tropical areas, but certain species are found as far north as Sweden and others as far south as Tasmania.

Older classifications referred to this genus under the name of *Taeniorhynchus*. Some modern classifications recognise *Mansonia* and *Coquillettidia* as distinct genera, but in the present book only one genus, *Mansonia*, is recognised. This genus (*Mansonia*) contains four subgenera, two of which, *Mansonioides* and *Coquillettidia*, contain most of the medically important species.

Eggs

Species belonging to the subgenus *Coquillettidia*, lay their eggs on the water surface in the form of egg rafts and look rather similar to those of *Culex* rafts. However, in *Coquillettidia* the eggs are often arranged in fewer rows so that elongated rafts are produced (Fig. 3.8) which can be distinguished from the less elongated *Culex* egg rafts (see Fig. 1.15). The individual eggs are

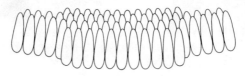

Fig. 3.8   Long and narrow egg raft, typical of *Mansonia* subgenus *Coquillettidia*.

cylindrical, brown or brownish-black. Egg rafts are found only in more or less permanent collections of water having rooted or free floating vegetation. Species of the subgenus *Mansonioides* lay their eggs in sticky compact masses, often arranged as circular rosettes, which are glued to the undersurfaces of floating vegetation (see Figs. 1.15 and 3.9). Individual eggs are dark brown-black and cylindrical, but with a tube-like extension apically which is usually darker than the rest of the egg.

Eggs of *Coquillettidia* and *Mansonioides* hatch within a few days. They cannot withstand desiccation.

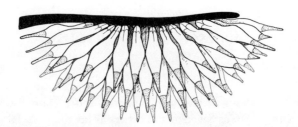

Fig. 3.9   Eggs of *Mansonia* subgenus *Mansonioides* glued to undersurface of floating vegetation.

Larvae

Larvae of the genus *Mansonia* are very easily recognised because they have specialised siphons adapted for piercing aquatic plants to obtain air (Fig. 3.10). The siphon is conical with the apical part dark and heavily sclerotised, it has prehensile hairs and serrated processes for inserting into plants.

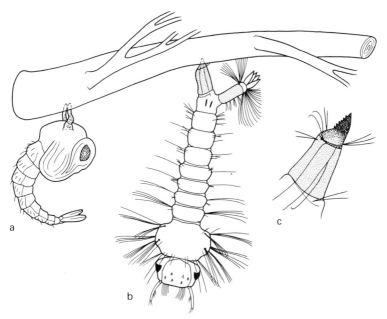

Fig. 3.10 Immature stages of *Mansonia* mosquitoes. (a) Pupa with respiratory trumpets inserted into an aquatic plant; (b) larva with siphon inserted into a plant for respiration; (c) larval siphon showing serrated structures.

Adults

Adults of most species belonging to the subgenus *Coquillettidia* are rather large and predominantly yellow, whereas those of the subgenus *Mansonioides* (which contains important filariasis vectors) are usually smaller and duller mosquitoes. Typically, they have the legs (Fig. 3.11c), palps, wings and body covered with a mixture of dark (usually brown) and pale (white or creamy) scales, giving the insect a rather dusty look. The speckled pattern of dark and pale scales on the wing veins, gives the wings the appearance

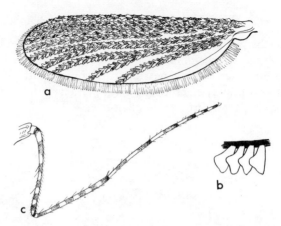

Fig. 3.11 *Mansonia* adult. (a) Wing showing 'salt and pepper'-like distribution of dark and pale scales on the wing veins; (b) a few wing scales showing their broad shape; (c) leg showing ring-like distribution dark and pale scales.

of having been sprinkled with salt and pepper (Fig. 3.11a), and provides a useful character for identifying the adults. Closer examination shows that the scales on the wing veins are very broad and often asymmetrical (Fig. 3.11b). In other mosquitoes these scales are longer and narrower.

Biology

Eggs are laid either in rafts floating on the water surface (subgenus *Coquillettidia*), or in egg masses glued to the undersurface of vegetation (subgenus *Mansonioides*); they hatch within a few days. All larval habitats have aquatic vegetation, either rooted, such as grasses, rushes and reeds, or floating, such as *Pistia stratiotes*, *Salvinia* and *Eichhornia*. Larvae consequently occur in permanent collections of water such as swamps, marshes, ponds, borrow pits, grassy ditches, irrigation canals and even in the middle of rivers if they have floating vegetation. Wherever the water lettuce, *Pistia stratiotes*, is present, breeding by *Mansonia* should be suspected.

Pupae have elongated and pointed respiratory trumpets which are modified for inserting into aquatic plants for respiration (Fig. 3.10a).

Larvae and pupae only detach themselves from plants and rise to the surface of the water if they are disturbed. Because they are more or less permanently attached to plants the immature stages are frequently missed in larval surveys. It is therefore not easy to identify breeding places with certainty unless special collecting procedures are undertaken, such as the collection of plants to which the immature stages are thought to be attached. It is often difficult to control breeding of *Mansonia* species by conventional insecticidal applications, because of the problems of getting the insecticides to the larvae, which may be some distance below the water surface (see p. 86).

Adults usually bite during the night, but some species are day-biters. After feeding most *Mansonia* rest out of doors, but a few species rest indoors. The important vector species belong to the subgenus *Mansonioides*. For example, *Ma. uniformis* which is a vector of nocturnal periodic *Brugia malayi* in the Indian sub-continent and South-east Asia, and also of *Wuchereria bancrofti* in New Guinea. *Mansonia annulifera, Ma. annulata* and *Ma. indiana*, are vectors of nocturnal subperiodic *B. malayi* in South-east Asia and sometimes also in the Indian subcontinent. In Africa, filariasis (*W. bancrofti*) is not transmitted by *Mansonia* species, but several species, especially *Ma. africana* and *Ma. uniformis*, are vectors of various arboviruses.

MEDICAL IMPORTANCE

Biting nuisance

In several areas of the world a lot of money is spent on mosquito control, not so much because mosquitoes are vectors of disease but because they are such troublesome biters. For example, some of the best organised mosquito control operations are in North America, where more money is spent on killing culicine mosquitoes than is expended in most tropical countries where they are important vectors of disease. In northern temperate and sub-arctic parts of America, Europe and Asia much greater numbers of *Aedes* mosquitoes can be encountered biting man than in tropical countries. Although they are not transmitting diseases to man in these areas they can, nevertheless, make life outdoors almost intolerable.

Yellow fever

The arbovirus causing yellow fever occurs in Africa and tropical areas of the Americas. It does not occur in Asia or elsewhere, although mosquitoes capable of transmitting the disease occur in many countries. Yellow fever is a zoonosis, being essentially a disease of forest monkeys which under certain conditions can be transmitted to man.

Africa

In Africa the yellow fever virus occurs in certain cercopithecid monkeys inhabiting the forests and is transmitted amongst them mainly by *Aedes africanus*. This is a forest dwelling mosquito that breeds in tree holes and bites mainly in the forest canopy soon after sunset—just in the right place at the right time to bite monkeys going to sleep in the tree tops. This sylvatic, forest or monkey cycle, as it is sometimes called, maintains a reservoir in the monkey population (Fig. 3.12). In Africa, monkeys are little affected by yellow fever, dying only occasionally. Some species of monkeys involved in the forest cycle, such as the red-tailed guenon, descend from the trees to steal bananas from farms at the edge of the forest. In this habitat the monkeys get bitten by different mosquitoes including *Aedes simpsoni*. This species bites during the day at the edge of forests and breeds in leaf axils of bananas, plantains and other plants such as *Colocasia* and pineapples. If the monkeys have viraemia, that is yellow fever virus circulating in their peripheral blood, *Ae. simpsoni* becomes infected, and if the mosquito lives long enough it can transmit yellow fever to other monkeys or more importantly to man. This transmission cycle, occurring in clearings at the edge of the forest involving monkeys, *Ae. simpsoni* and man, is sometimes referred to as the rural cycle (Fig. 3.12). When man returns to his village or travels to towns he is bitten by different mosquitoes, including *Ae. aegypti*, a domestic species breeding mainly in man-made containers such as water-storage pots, abandoned tin cans and vehicle tyres. If man is showing viraemia *Ae. aegypti* becomes infected and yellow fever is then transmitted amongst the human population by this species. This is the urban cycle of yellow fever transmission (Fig. 3.12).

It is possible for man to become infected in the forest by bites

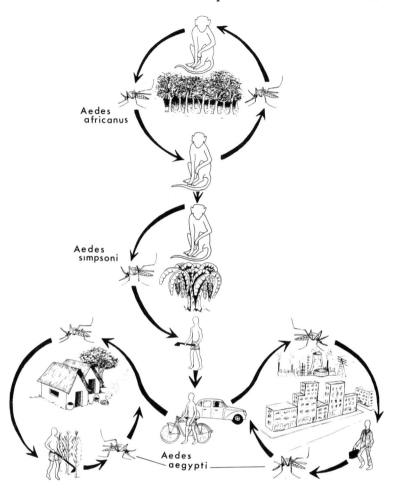

Fig. 3.12 Diagrammatic representation of the sylvatic, rural and urban transmission cycles of yellow fever in Africa.

of *Ae. africanus*, but the likelihood of man acquiring yellow fever by a canopy feeding mosquito is remote. The epidemiology of yellow fever is complicated by differences in the feeding behaviour of different populations of *Ae. aegypti*, and more especially *Ae. simpsoni*. In some areas for example, yellow fever may be circulating amongst the monkey population yet rarely get transmitted to man because local populations of *Ae. simpsoni* are predominantly zoophagic. Other primates in Africa such as *Galago* species may also be reservoirs of yellow fever.

Americas

In Central and South America the yellow fever cycle, although similar to that in Africa, differs in certain aspects (Fig. 3.13). As in Africa it is a disease of forest monkeys, mainly cebid ones, and it is transmitted amongst them by forest dwelling mosquitoes. The most important vectors are *Haemagogus spegazzinii, Hg. equinus, Hg. janthinomys* (=*falco*), *Hg. leucocelaenus* and *Sabethes chloropterus*, although this last species appears to be an inefficient vector. These are arboreal mosquitoes which bite in the forest

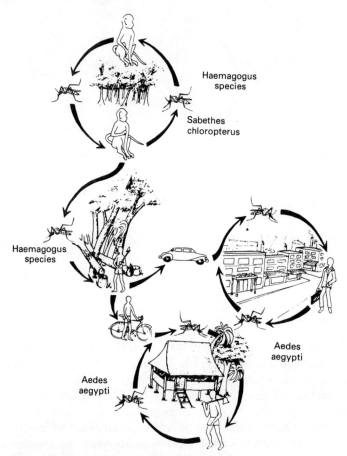

Fig. 3.13 Diagrammatic representation of the jungle, rural and urban transmission cycles of yellow fever in Central and South America.

canopy and breed in tree holes. New World monkeys are more susceptible to yellow fever than African monkeys and they frequently become sick and die. When people enter the jungle to cut down trees for timber, mosquitoes, which normally bite monkeys at canopy height, may descend and bite man; if they are infected man develops yellow fever. The disease is then spread from man to man in villages and towns, as in Africa, by *Ae. aegypti* (Fig. 3.13). It is possible that in South America marsupials and even sloths and porcupines may be involved in yellow fever cycles.

Viraemia

The intrinsic incubation period of yellow fever in man is about 4–5 days, usually a little less in monkeys. Thus, after 4 or 5 days the virus appears in the peripheral blood, that is viraemia is produced, and this occurs irrespectively of whether monkeys or man are showing overt symptoms of the disease. Viraemia lasts only 2 days, after which the virus disappears from the peripheral blood never to return and the individual is immune. Monkeys and man are therefore infective to mosquitoes for only about 2 days in their entire lives. A relatively high titre of yellow fever (and also any other arbovirus) is needed before it can pass across the gut cells of the mosquito into the haemolymph, from which it invades many tissues and organs, including the salivary glands, where virus multiplication occurs. This is the extrinsic cycle of development and takes 5–30 days, depending on temperature, the type of arbovirus and mosquito host. A mosquito must therefore live for a sufficiently long time before it becomes infective and capable of transmitting yellow fever, or any other virus. Recently it has been shown that infected *Aedes* mosquitoes can pass on yellow fever virus through their progeny, so that the next generation of adults are already infected, even before they have bitten a host. This is an example of transovarial transmission, a phenomenon more usually associated with tick-borne viruses. The importance of transovarial yellow fever transmission is not yet determined.

Mosquito dissections cannot show whether mosquitoes are infected with yellow fever, or any other virus. To determine whether they are infected with arboviruses several female mosquitoes are ground up and inoculated into young mice or other susceptible hosts. After an incubation period any viruses developing in these hosts are passaged to others. Arbovirus isolations and identifications are usually carried out in specially equipped virology laboratories.

Dengue

A number of different viruses (dengue types 1, 2, 3, 4, and ?5) are responsible for true dengue. This disease (or diseases) was first reported in epidemic form in India and Java, but now occurs in many areas of the world including southern USA, West Indies, Central and South America, Greece, West and East Africa, South-east Asia, Hawaii and Australia. More recently a more severe form, which tends to cause infant mortality (haemorrhagic dengue), has appeared in many areas of South-east Asia, such as Thailand, Malaysia, Laos, the Philippines, and also India. In 1981 haemorrhagic dengue and dengue type 4 were first noticed in the Caribbean.

Both the classical and haemorrhagic forms are transmitted principally by *Ae. aegypti*; in South-east Asia *Ae. albopictus*, and in Uganda *Ae. simpsoni* are less important vectors. Mosquitoes of the *Ae. scutellaris* group may also transmit dengue in the Pacific islands and New Guinea. There are no known animal reservoirs, but it is possible that monkeys and other primates might be involved.

The encephalitis viruses

Several viruses transmitted by mosquitoes, predominantly in the Americas but also elsewhere, are included in this category; for example, Eastern equine encephalitis (EEE), Western equine encephalitis (WEE), Venezuelan equine encephalitis (VEE), St Louis encephalitis (SLE) and Japanese encephalitis (JE). All these viruses involve a zoonosis with birds, especially herons and passerines which feed and/or nest near marshes. The three equine encephalitis viruses are very virulent in horses as well as man. These diseases are sometimes referred to as encephalomyelites viruses and sometimes the word equine is omitted from their names, for example VEE may be called Venezuelan encephalitis.

Eastern equine encephalitis occurs mainly in the eastern area of the USA, but extends down into South America. It is also found in parts of Asia, Europe and Australasia. EEV is principally a disease of birds, and in North America it is spread mainly by *Culiseta melanura* (the genus *Culiseta* is not discussed in this book), and *Mansonia perturbans*. It is transmitted to man and horses, and sometimes also birds, by various *Aedes* species.

Western equine and St Louis encephalitis viruses are widely distributed in the USA and extend into northern parts of South America. They are basically arboviruses infecting birds and are transmitted principally by *Culex tarsalis*, a rice field breeding mosquito, other *Culex* mosquitoes and *Culiseta inornata*. These mosquitoes transmit the disease to birds and also to man and horses. In towns SLE infects not only wild birds but also poultry and is spread by several *Culex* species including *Cx. nigripalpus* and *Cx. pipiens*. Bats may also be involved in the zoonotic cycle.

Venezuelan equine encephalitis virus is probably the most important of these encephalitis viruses. It is found in southern USA through Central to South America and is transmitted amongst birds, and occasionally bats, by several *Culex* and *Aedes* mosquitoes. In Central and South America the virus also occurs in forest rodents, marsupials and monkeys. Man and horses become infected. Other mosquito genera, especially *Mansonia* species, have been incriminated in spreading VEE.

Japanese encephalitis occurs not only in Japan but in India, China, Malaysia, Korea and other areas of South-east Asia. The basic transmission cycle involves birds, mainly herons, egrets and ibises. Pigs, however, are also important reservoir hosts particularly in warm areas where they develop high viraemias, and are called amplifying hosts. Transmission to birds, man and pigs is mainly by *Cx. tritaeniorhynchus* which is a very common rice field breeding mosquito. *Culex gelidus* probably maintains the virus in pig-to-pig transmission. Bats also become infected, and may play a role in transmission.

All these encephalitic viruses have a more complex epidemiology than described here, involving several different transmission cycles having different animal reservoirs and mosquito vectors.

The viraemia produced in man by VEE, SLE, JE and EEE, and sometimes also by WEE, is so low that the disease cannot be transmitted from man to man or from man to any other susceptible hosts by mosquitoes. Thus man is a 'dead-end' host and horses are similarly 'dead-end' hosts for the encephalitis viruses infecting them.

Other arboviruses

There are many other arboviruses transmitted to man by mosquitoes, such as Chikungunya (CHIK) in East Africa and India; West Nile (WN) in Africa, Europe, Israel and Asia; Bunyamwere (BUN) in Africa; Ilheus (ILH) in Brazil, Trinidad and Panama; and Murray Valley encephalitis (MVE) in Australia. A few mosquito-borne arboviruses are found in Europe as far west as France, but there is no evidence that any arboviruses are transmitted by mosquitoes in Britain. Some arboviruses are transmitted by genera of mosquitoes not referred to in this book.

Transovarial transmission is sometimes an important phenomenon with rickettsiae and arboviruses infecting ticks and mites (Chapters 17 and 19), but until comparatively recently was unknown in mosquitoes. However, it is now known that certain arboviruses (e.g. yellow fever) can invade the ovaries of mosquitoes and infect the next generation. But with many viruses the importance of such transovarial transmission remains unclear.

Filariasis (Table 3.1)

The development of filarial worms in mosquito vectors is briefly described in the preceding chapter (p. 53).

Bancroftian filariasis

Wuchereria bancrofti occurs throughout the tropics and also in certain subtropical areas. It is essentially an urban disease, there are no animal reservoirs and the parasites can develop only in man and mosquitoes.

The **nocturnal periodic** form of *Wuchereria bancrofti* is transmitted both by various *Anopheles* species (Chapter 2) and, throughout much of its distribution, also by *Culex quinquefasciatus*. This mosquito is widespread in the tropics and breeds mainly in man-made containers and polluted waters such as septic tanks, cess pits, drains and ditches, pots and water-storage jars, especially those organically polluted. It is a mosquito that has increased in many towns due to increasing urbanisation and the resultant proliferation of insanitary collections of water. It is principally a night biter. After feeding adults may rest in houses. In New Guinea *Mansonia uniformis* and night biting *Culex* species

Table 3.1 Summary of principal mosquito vectors of filariasis.

Species and forms of filariasis	Geographic distribution	Vectors	Zoonotic reservoir
Wuchereria bancrofti			
Nocturnal periodic	Throughout tropics (but not Polynesia)	*Anopheles* spp., including many malaria vectors of different areas	None
	Throughout tropics (but not Polynesia)	*Culex quinquefasciatus*	
	New Guinea	*Mansonia uniformis*	
	China and Japan	*Aedes togoi*	
	Philippines	*Aedes poicilius*	
Diurnal subperiodic	Polynesia	*Aedes polynesiensis*	None
	Fiji	*Aedes pseudoscutellaris*	
	New Caledonia	*Aedes vigilax*	
Nocturnal subperiodic	Thailand	*Aedes niveus* group	None
Brugia malayi			
Nocturnal periodic (principally open swamps)	Asia, from India to Japan	*Anopheles* spp., including many malaria vectors of different areas	Not important, possibly some exist
	Asia, from India to Japan	*Mansonia annulifera, Ma. uniformis, Ma. indiana*, etc.	
	China, Korea and Japan	*Aedes togoi*	
Nocturnal subperiodic (mainly in swampy forests)	Malaysia, Brunei, Philippines, Thailand, Vietnam	*Mansonia dives, Ma. bonneae, Ma. annulata, Ma. uniformis*, etc.	Monkeys, especially leaf-monkeys (*Presbytis* spp.), civet cats and pangolins
Brugia timori			
Nocturnal periodic	Timor, Flores and Alor islands in Indonesia	*Anopheles* spp. of the *barbirostris* group	None

are also vectors of *W. bancrofti*, but in contrast *Mansonia* species do not transmit filariasis in Africa.

In Japan and China, *Aedes togoi*, which breeds in rock pools containing brackish water and in rain-filled receptacles such as pots and cisterns, is also a vector of nocturnal periodic bancroftian filariasis, although it is more usually thought of as being a vector of brugian filariasis. It bites man early in the evenings around sunset. In the Philippines *Aedes poicilius* is the most important vector of nocturnal periodic *W. bancrofti*. Larvae occur in leaf axils of banana, plantain and *Colocasia* plants. Adults bite in the early part of the night, mainly indoors but also sometimes outdoors. Adults rest outdoors after feeding.

The **diurnal subperiodic** form of *W. bancrofti* occurs in Polynesia where the nocturnal periodic form is absent. The most important vector is *Ae. polynesiensis*, a day-biting mosquito which feeds mostly outdoors but may enter houses to bite; adults rest almost exclusively outdoors. Larvae occur in natural containers such as split coconut shells, leaf bracts and crab holes, and also in man-made containers such as discarded tins, pots, vehicle tyres, canoes and drums. *Aedes pseudoscutellaris* is another outdoor day-biting mosquito that is a vector of diurnal subperiodic *bancrofti* in Fiji. It breeds mainly in tree holes and bamboo stumps but larvae are also found in crab holes. In New Caledonia *Ae. polynesiensis* is absent and *Ae. vigilax*, which breeds in brackish or fresh water in rock pools and ground pools, is the most important vector. Adults rest and feed outdoors, mainly during the day.

In Thailand a nocturnal subperiodic form of *W. bancrofti* occurs that is transmitted by the *Ae. niveus* group of mosquitoes.

It should be noted that although several *Aedes* mosquitoes are vectors of filariasis, especially the bancroftian form, *Ae. aegypti* is not a vector of filariasis to man.

Natural infection rates of mosquitoes with infective larvae of *W. bancrofti* vary from about 0·1–5 per cent, depending greatly on the vector species and local conditions.

Brugian filariasis

The **nocturnal periodic** form of *Brugia malayi* occurs throughout most of Asia, from India, Sri Lanka, Malaysia, Indonesia, Borneo, China to parts of Japan. There do not appear to be any important animal reservoirs, although possibly cats may be infected. It is transmitted mainly by night-biting *Mansonia* mosquitoes, such as *Ma. indiana*, *Ma. annulifera*, *Ma. uniformis* and also various *Anopheles* species (Chapter 2). These *Mansonia* species breed in more or less permanent collections of water with floating or rooted vegetation, such as swamps and ponds. Adults bite man mainly outdoors and rest out of doors afterwards, but they will also bite and rest indoors in some areas. In China, Korea and Japan *Ae. togoi* is a vector of nocturnal periodic *B. malayi*.

The **nocturnal subperiodic** form of *B. malayi* occurs in Malaysia, Brunei, Thailand, Vietnam and the Philippines and is transmitted by *Mansonia* mosquitoes, mainly by *Ma. annulata*, *Ma. dives*, *Ma. bonneae* and *Ma. uniformis*. Larvae occur in habitats with much vegetation, such as swampy forests. Adults bite mainly at night but also during the daytime, especially species such as *Ma. dives* and *Ma. bonneae*. The subperiodic form of *B. malayi* is essentially a disease of swamp monkeys, especially the leaf monkeys (*Presbytis* spp.), but domestic and wild cats, such as civet cats, and pangolins appear to be minor reservoirs of infection.

Natural infection rates of mosquitoes with infective larvae of *B. malayi* range from about 0·1 to 2 or 3 per cent, which is slightly lower than with *W. bancrofti*, but these vary according to mosquito species and local conditions.

As mentioned in Chapter 2, the discovery of filarial worms in mosquitoes does not necessarily imply that they are vectors of either *W. bancrofti* or *B. malayi* because mosquitoes are also vectors of several other filarial parasites of animals.

CONTROL

The use of suitable repellents, mosquito nets and mosquito screening of houses and other personal protection measures (discussed in Chapters 1 and 2), can give some relief from culicine mosquitoes. It is, however, often more difficult to obtain protection from culicines than anophelines because many of them bite outdoors during the daytime. Spraying the interior surfaces of houses with residual insecticides, as practised for *Anopheles* control, is not usually applicable to culicines, because most species do not rest predominantly in houses. The main method of attack involves larval control, although sometimes aerial ULV applications are used to kill adult culicine mosquitoes.

Control measures against *Ae. aegypti*, *Ae. polynesiensis* and *Ae. albopictus*, species which breed mainly in man-made containers in both rural and urban areas, are often aimed at reducing the numbers of larval habitats, that is control by source reduction. Thus, people are encouraged not to store water in pots inside or outside houses, or allow water to accumulate in discarded tin cans, bottles, vehicle tyres, etc. However, persuading people to cooperate in reducing peridomestic breeding of these vectors is often unsuccessful unless local legislation is strictly enforced. A reliable piped water supply to houses can do much to reduce *Ae. aegypti* breeding.

In situations where source reduction is not feasible, insecticidal applications to breeding sites can be attempted. Although insecticidal spraying will kill *Aedes* larvae it usually has no effect on their dry, but viable, eggs. These have been deposited at the edges of larval habitats and will hatch when the water level rises and floods them. *Aedes* mosquitoes breeding in pools, ponds and marshy areas can be controlled by ground-based or aerial applications of granular organophosphate insecticides. Applications can be made either before or after habitats have become flooded, that is pre- or post-flood treatments. Insecticidal granules landing on dry or muddy grounds remain more or less inactive until the habitats become flooded. When this occurs previously dry aedine eggs hatch, but at the same time flooding results in the release of insecticide from the granules and this kills the newly hatched larvae. This technique helps to overcome the problem of controlling *Aedes* mosquitoes whose eggs may hatch in instalments over extended periods after flooding. The more persistent the insecticides incorporated in these granules or pellets the longer effective control can be achieved. Organochlorine insecticides are very persistent but they are not recommended for larval control because they are, in fact, too persistent and not biodegradable. As a consequence their residues accumulate in food chains and cause ecological damage. Consequently, most granular preparations used to control *Aedes* larvae are formulated from organophosphates, such as chlorpyrifos (Dursban) and temephos (Abate).

When insecticides are applied to kill mosquitoes breeding in water used for drinking, it is essential that they have extremely low mammalian toxicity and impart no taste or odour to the water. The insecticide that can safely be recommended for treating such water is temephos. Granular formulations of this insecticide can remain effective in killing *Ae. aegypti* larvae for about 5 weeks after their application.

In most countries *Ae. aegypti* has developed insecticide resistance to DDT, dieldrin and HCH, and also to various organophosphate insecticides. In Thailand *Ae. aegypti* is resistant to the synthetic pyrethroid, bioresmethrin. Insecticides that are commonly used for larval control of *Ae. aegypti* include temephos (Abate), chlorpyrifos (Dursban), fenthion (Baytex), malathion and carbaryl (Sevin).

Ground-based or aerial ULV applications of insecticides such as malathion, chlorpyrifos (Dursban), propoxur (Baygon), fenitrothion (Sumithion) and synthetic pyrethroids have been used to kill adult *Ae. aegypti*. Aeroplane ULV spraying has, on several occasions, helped to control *Ae. aegypti* during dengue outbreaks. In emergencies such as dengue or yellow fever epidemics several control methods are usually employed simultaneously to kill the vectors.

Culex quinquefasciatus, an important filariasis vector, is best controlled by improving sanitation and installing modern sewage systems, but often this is not feasible and insecticidal measures have to be employed. In most areas *Cx. quinquefasciatus* is resistant to the organochlorine insecticides, also in many areas to the organophophate compounds and in the USA to propoxur. This consequently limits the insecticides than can be effectively used. Larval habitats should be sprayed weekly. Usually, relatively large dosage rates have to be applied because most insecticides are less effective in the presence of organic pollution, which is characteristic of most *Cx. quinquefasciatus* breeding places. In the USA aerial ULV spraying has frequently been used against various vectors of the encephalitis viruses. Some important encephalitis vectors, such as *Cx. tarsalis* in the USA and *Cx. tritaeniorhynchus* in many parts of Asia, have become resistant to DDT, dieldrin and HCH and in addition several organophosphate compounds.

Mansonia mosquitoes are usually controlled by removing or killing the aquatic weeds upon which the larvae and pupae depend for their oxygen requirements. Weeds such as *Pistia stratiotes* can sometimes be removed manually from small areas such as borrow pits. Alternatively they can be sprayed with herbicides, such as paraquat, diquat, 2,4-dichlorophenoxyacetic acid (2,4-D), dichlobenil, 4-chloro-2-methylphenoxyacetic acid (MCPA) or pentachlorophenol (PCP). The last herbicide has proved exceptionally good at killing *Salvinia*, an aquatic weed frequently associated with *Mansonia* breeding. Altering aquatic habitats by the removal or destruction of weeds may result in ecological changes that allow the habitat to be colonised by mosquito species that were previously excluded by the dense covering of weeds.

If insecticides are used to control *Mansonia* larvae, then granules or pellets are more suitable than liquid formulations. This is because they can penetrate the vegetation, sink to the bottom of breeding places and release their chemicals through the water. However, species such as *Ma. dives* and *Ma. bonneae*, which are important vectors of brugian filariasis, breed in extensive swampy forests, and are impossible to control because of the large and often inaccessible areas involved.

The spread of insecticide resistance amongst many culicine vectors has caused renewed interest in some of the older control methods, such as the use of high spreading oils and granular preparations of Paris green.

Chapter 4
Blackflies

Blackflies have a world-wide distribution. There are nearly 1300 species in some 12 genera. However, only four genera, *Simulium*, *Prosimulium*, *Austrosimulium* and *Cnephia*, contain regular man-biting species.

Medically, *Simulium* is by far the most important genus as it contains important vector species. In Africa, *S. damnosum** and *S. neavei*, and in Central and Southern America, *As. ochraceum* and *S. metallicum*, transmit the parasitic nematode *Onchocerca volvulus* to man, which causes onchocerciasis (river blindness). In Brazil *S. amazonicum* has been found infected with *Mansonella ozzardi*, a filarial parasite that is usually regarded as non-pathogenic.

EXTERNAL MORPHOLOGY

The Simuliidae are commonly known as blackflies, but in some areas, in particular Australia, they may be called sandflies. As explained in Chapter 5 this latter terminology is confusing and best avoided because biting flies of the family Ceratopogonidae, and flies of the subfamily Phlebotominae are also called sandflies.

Adult blackflies are quite small, about 1·5–4 mm long, relatively stout-bodied and, when viewed from the side, have a rather humped thorax. As their vernacular name indicates they are usually black in colour but many have contrasting patterns of white, silvery or yellowish hairs on their bodies and legs, while others may be predominantly or largely orange or bright yellow.

Blackflies have a pair of large compound eyes, which in females

---

* Formerly regarded as a single species, but cytotaxonomic studies reveal that there are about 27 distinct species or cytotypes within the *S. damnosum* complex. They differ in their distribution, ecology and behaviour; fortunately not all species are vectors of onchocerciasis.

are separated on the top of the head (a condition known as dichoptic); in the males the eyes occupy almost all of the head and
touch on top of it and in front, above the bases of the antennae
(a condition known as holoptic) (Fig. 4.1). The antennae are short
and stout, distinctly segmented but without long hairs. The
mouthparts are short and relatively inconspicuous but the five-
segmented maxillary palps, which arise at their base, hang downwards and are easily seen. Only females bite. The arrangement
and morphology of the mouthparts is similar to those of the biting
midges (Ceratopogonidae, Chapter 6). The mouthparts, being
short and broad, do not penetrate very deeply into the host's
tissues. Teeth on the labrum stretch the skin, and the rasp-like

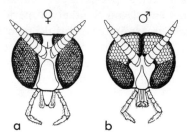

Fig. 4.1 Front view of simuliid heads. (a) adult female with dichoptic eyes; (b)
adult male with holoptic eyes.

action of the maxillae and mandibles cuts through it and ruptures
the fine blood capillaries. The small pool of blood produced is
then sucked up by the flies. This method of feeding is ideally
suited for picking up the microfilariae of *Onchocerca volvulus*
which occur in man's skin not blood.

The thorax is covered dorsally with very fine and appressed
hairs, which can be black, white, silvery, yellow or orange and
may be arranged in various patterns. The relatively short legs are
also covered with very fine and closely appressed hairs and may
be uni-colorous or have contrasting bands of pale and dark colour.
The wings are characteristically short and broad and lack scales
or prominent hairs. Only the veins near the anterior margin are
well developed, the rest of the wing is membraneous and has an
indistinct venation (Fig. 4.2). The wings are colourless or almost
so. When at rest the wings are closed flat over the body like the
blades of a closed pair of scissors.

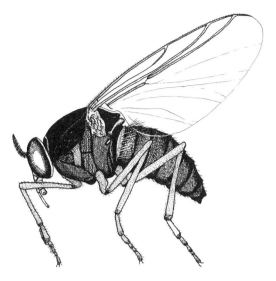

Fig. 4.2 Simuliid blackfly adult.

The abdomen is short and squat, and covered with inconspicuous closely appressed fine hairs. In neither sex are the genitalia very conspicuous. Blackflies are most easily sexed by looking at the eyes.

THE LIFE-CYCLE

When first laid the eggs are pale and often whitish but darken to a brown or black colour. They are about 0·1–0·4 mm long, more or less triangular in shape but with rounded corners and have smooth unsculptured shells (Fig. 4.3a) which are covered with a sticky substance. They are always laid in flowing water but the type of breeding place differs greatly according to species. Habitats can vary from small trickles of water, slow flowing streams, lake outlets and water flowing from dams to fast flowing rivers and rapids. Some species prefer lowland streams and rivers while others are found in mountain rivers. In species such as *S. ochraceum*, one of the South American vectors of onchocerciasis, eggs are scattered over the surface of flowing water while females are in flight. In most species, however, ovipositing females alight on partially immersed objects such as rocks, stones and vegetation,

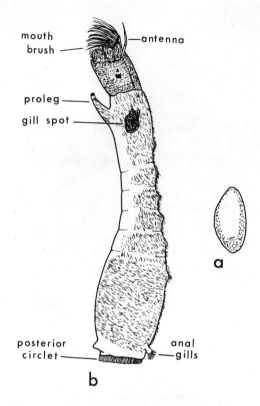

mouth
brush —————— antenna

proleg ————

gill spot ————

a

posterior   anal
circlet ————   —gills

b

Fig. 4.3   (a) Simuliid egg; (b) last instar larva of a simuliid species of the *Simulium damnosum* complex, showing body covered in minute dark setae and dorsal tubercles.

to lay their eggs. Usually some 150–800 eggs are laid in sticky masses or strings on a level with, or just below the water line on submerged objects. Females may crawl underneath the water and become completely submerged during oviposition. There may be a few favoured oviposition sites in a stream or river, resulting in thousands of eggs from many females being found together. *Simulium damnosum*, for example, frequently has such communal oviposition sites.

Eggs of *S. damnosum* hatch within about 1 day but in many other tropical species the egg stage lasts 2–4 days. Eggs of species inhabiting temperate and cold northern areas may not hatch for many weeks and some species pass the winter as diapausing eggs.

There are 6–8 larval instars and the mature larva is about 5–13 mm long, depending on the species, and easily distinguished from all other aquatic larvae (Fig. 4.3b). The head is usually black, or almost so, and has a prominent pair of feeding brushes (cephalic fans), while the weakly segmented, cylindrical body is usually whitish, but may be darker or sometimes even greenish. The body is slightly swollen beyond the head and in most, but not all, species distinctly swollen towards the end. The rectum has finger-like gills which on larval preservation may be extruded and visible as a protuberance from the dorsal surface towards the end of the abdomen. Ventrally, just below the head, is a small pseudopod called the proleg which is armed with small circles of hooklets.

Larvae do not swim but remain sedentary for long periods on submerged vegetation, rocks, stones and other debris. Attachment is achieved by the posterior hook-circlet (anal sucker of many previous authors) tightly gripping a small silken pad. This has been produced by the larva's very large salivary glands and is firmly glued to the substrate. Larvae can nevertheless move about and change their position. This is achieved by alternately attaching themselves to the substrate by the proleg and the posterior hook-circlet, thus they move in a looping manner. When larvae are disturbed they can deposit sticky saliva on a submerged object, release their hold and be swept downstream for some distance at the end of a silken thread. They can then either swallow the thread of saliva and regain their original position, or reattach themselves at sites further downstream. Larvae normally orientate themselves to lie parallel to the flow of water with their heads downstream. They are mainly filter-feeders, ingesting, with the aid of large mouth brushes, suspended particles of food. However, a few species have predacious larvae and others are occasionally cannibalistic. Larval development may be as short as 1–2 weeks, depending on species and temperature, and in some species may be extended to several months, in other species larvae overwinter.

Mature larvae, which can be recognised by a blackish mark termed the gill spot (respiratory organ of the future pupa), on each side of the thorax (Fig. 4.3b), spin, with the silk produced by the salivary glands, a protective slipper-shaped brownish cocoon. This cocoon is firmly stuck to submerged vegetation, rocks or other objects (Fig. 4.4) and its shape and structure vary greatly according to species. After weaving the cocoon the enclosed larva pupates. The pupa has a pair of, usually prominent, filamentous or broad thin-walled, respiratory gills. Their length, shape and the number of filaments or branches provide useful taxonomic characters for species identification. These gills, and the anterior part of the pupa, often project from the entrance of the cocoon (Fig. 4.4). In both tropical and non-tropical countries the pupal period lasts only 2–6 days and is unusual in not appearing to be

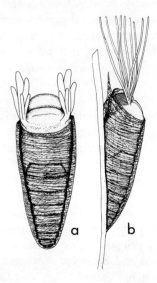

Fig. 4.4 Simuliid pupae. (a) dorsal view of species with broad and short respiratory filaments; (b) lateral view of species with long filamentous respiratory filaments.

dependent on temperature. On emergence adults either rise rapidly to the water surface in a protective bubble of gas, which prevents them from being wetted, or they escape by crawling up partially submerged objects such as vegetation or rocks. A characteristic of many species is the more or less simultaneous mass emergence of thousands of adults. On reaching the water surface the adults immediately take flight.

The empty pupal cases, with gill filaments still attached, remain enclosed in their cocoons after the adults have emerged and retain their taxonomic value. Consequently, they provide useful information on the species of simuliids that have recently bred and successfully emerged from various habitats.

A few African blackfly species, such as *S. neavei*, have a very unusual aquatic existence. Their larvae (except the 1st-instar) and pupae do not occur on submerged rocks or vegetation but on other aquatic arthropods, such as the bodies of immature stages (nymphs) of mayflies (Ephemeroptera), and various crustacea including fresh water crabs. Such an association is termed a phoretic relationship. Eggs, however, are never found on these animals; they are probably laid on submerged stones or vegetation (see also p. 96).

Adult behaviour

Both male and female blackflies feed on plant juices and naturally occurring sugary substances, but only females take blood-meals. Biting occurs out of doors at almost any daylight hour, but each species may have its preferred times of biting. For example, in Africa *S. damnosum* has a biting peak in the morning and another in the afternoon, whereas in South America *S. ochraceum* bites predominantly early in the morning between 08.00–10.00 h. Many species seem particularly active on cloudy, overcast days and in thundery weather. Species may exhibit marked preferences for feeding on different parts of the body, for example, *S. damnosum* feeds mainly on the legs whereas *S. ochraceum* prefers to bite the upper part of the body. When feeding on animals, adults crawl down the fur of mammals, or feathers of birds, to bite the host's skin, they may also enter the ears to feed.

Many species of blackfly feed almost exclusively on birds (ornithophagic) and others on non-human mammalian hosts (zoophagic). However, several species also bite man. Some man-biting species seem to prefer various large animals such as donkeys or cattle and bite man only as a poor second choice, while others appear to find man an almost equally attractive host; no species bites man alone. In many species sight seems important in host location but host odours may also be important. After feeding, blood-engorged females shelter and rest in vegetation, on trees and in other natural out of door resting places until the blood-meal is completely digested. In the tropics this takes 2–3 days, in non–tropical areas it may take 3–8 days or longer, the speed of digestion depending mainly on temperature. Relatively little is known about blackfly longevity, but it seems that adults of most species live for 2–3 weeks, but some individuals may live as long as about 3 months.

Female blackflies may fly considerable distances from their emergence sites to obtain blood-meals and may also be dispersed large distances by winds. For example, it is not exceptional for adults of *S. damnosum* to be found biting 60–100 km from their breeding places. *S. damnosum* can be dispersed on prevailing winds as far as 300 km or possibly even 500 km. The long distances involved in dispersal have great relevance in control programmes because areas freed from blackflies can be reinvaded from distant breeding sites.

In temperate and northern areas of the Palearctic and Nearctic regions biting nuisance from simuliids is seasonal, because adults die in the autumn and new generations do not appear until the following spring or early summer. Although in many tropical areas there is continuous breeding throughout the year, there may nevertheless be dramatic increases in population size during the rainy season.

MEDICAL IMPORTANCE

Annoyance

In both tropical and non-tropical areas of the world blackflies can cause a very serious biting problem, since their bites can be painful. Although the severity of the reaction to bites differs in different individuals, localised swelling and inflammation frequently occurs, accompanied by intense irritation lasting for several days or even weeks. A form of dermatitis following the bites of *S. erythrocephalum* has been reported in Central Europe, and in the USA biting by *S. jenningsi* is said to have caused asthma. The classical example of the nuisance that can result from blackflies was the seasonal exodus during the 18th century, of people from the Danube valley areas in Central Europe, largely to save their domestic animals from attack by the enormous numbers of *S. colombaschense*. In some areas, such as northern territories of Canada, out of door activities are almost impossible at certain times of the year due to the intolerable numbers of biting simuliids. However, it is as disease vectors that blackflies are most important.

Onchocerciasis

The causative agent of human onchocerciasis, *Onchocerca volvulus*, or a morphologically very similar species, has been found in a monkey in Mexico and a gorilla in the Congo, but despite these discoveries and the fact that chimpanzees can be experimentally infected, there is no evidence that onchocerciasis is a zoonosis. The disease, commonly called river blindness, occurs throughout West Africa, Central Africa and much of East Africa between latitudes of approximately 15° north to 13° south, the most heavily infected areas being savanna regions, especially those in West Africa. A small focus is present in south Yemen and an autochthonous case has been reported from Saudi Arabia. The same parasite causes onchocerciasis in small localised areas in Central and South America, such as in southern Mexico, Guatemala, Brazil, Venezuela, Ecuador and Colombia.

Blackflies are the only vectors of human onchocerciasis. Their habit of tearing and rasping the skin to rupture the blood capillaries when obtaining a blood-meal makes them particularly suited to the ingestion of the skin-borne microfilariae of *O. volvulus*. Many of the microfilariae ingested during feeding are destroyed or excreted, but some penetrate the stomach wall and migrate to the thoracic muscles where they develop into sausage-shaped stages and undergo two moults. A few survive and elongate into thinner worms which pass through the head and down the short proboscis. The infective stages (about $550 \mu m$ in length) in the proboscis penetrate the host's skin when females alight to feed. The interval between the ingestion of microfilariae to the time infective larvae are in the proboscis is about 6–13 days, depending on temperature.

African vectors of onchocerciasis

Cytological studies have shown that the *S. damnosum* complex is composed of at least 27 distinct taxonomic forms, variously regarded as species or cytotypes. The *damnosum* complex is widespread in tropical Africa and certain members of the complex are the most important vectors of onchocerciasis in Africa.

Adults of the *damnosum* complex are mainly black. They can be recognised by the front tarsi being broad and flattened, having a conspicuous dorsal crest of fine hairs and by the presence of a very broad white area on the 1st segment of the hind tarsus (basitarsus). Larvae are found in the rapids of small or very large rivers in both savanna and forested areas of Africa. Adults frequently disperse far from their breeding sites and biting females can be encountered up to 100–250 km, or even 500 km away.

The other, but less important, African vector is *S. neavei*. This species is responsible for the transmission of onchocerciasis in both of the Congo Republics and Uganda, and formerly in Kenya where it is considered to have been eradicated by insecticidal control measures and bush clearing. It is a phoretic species, that is the larvae and pupae are found attached to other fresh water fauna, in this instance to crabs of the genus *Potamonautes* which occur in small rocky, rather turbid, streams and rivers.

American vectors of onchocerciasis

S. ochraceum is the principal onchocerciasis vector in southern Mexico and Guatemala, and is widely distributed in Central America and northern parts of South America. Adults are very small and are easily recognised by their dark brown legs, bright orange scutum and the yellow basal part of the abdomen, which contrasts with the black apical part. Females oviposit while in flight, dropping their eggs onto floating vegetation. Larval habitats consist of trickles of flowing water and very small streams which are often concealed by bushes, vegetation and fallen leaves. Adults do not appear to disperse far. The main biting season is unusual in being in the drier months of the year.

Simulium metallicum occurs in Mexico through Central America to northern areas of South America. In Venezuela it appears to be the most important vector while in other areas such as in Mexico and Guatemala it is considered a minor vector. It is a black species and has a broad white area on the first segment of the hind tarsus. Larvae occur in small or large streams and rivers. Adults fly further from their breeding sites than do those of *S. ochraceum*.

Other species known, or considered, to be local vectors of onchocerciasis in the Americas include *S. callidum* and *S. exiguum*.

Mansonella ozzardi

Mansonella ozzardi is a filarial parasite of man that is usually regarded as non-pathogenic, although it has been reported as causing morbidity in Colombia and Brazil. It is transmitted in Central and South America by *Culicoides* species (Chapter 5), but in Brazil *S. amazonicum* has been found to be infected.

CONTROL

There are few reports on the effectiveness of repellents against blackfly attacks. It seems that some protection, usually lasting up to 2 h, can be gained by use of repellents such as diethyltomuamide (DET), dimethyl phthalate (DMP) and butyryl-tetrahaydo quinoline.

Although insecticidal fogging or spraying of vegetation thought to harbour resting adult blackflies has occasionally been undertaken, this approach results in very temporary and localised control. The only practical method at present available for the control of blackflies is the application of insecticides to their breeding places to kill the larvae. Organochlorine or organophosphate insecticides need to be applied to only a few selected sites on watercourses for some 15–30 min, because as the insecticide is carried downstream it kills simuliid larvae over long stretches of water.The flow rates of the water and its depth are used to calculate the quantity of insecticide to be released. Applying DDT by this method has resulted in good control of *S. damnosum* in areas of Nigeria and Uganda. If treatment is not repeated at intervals throughout the year, gravid female adults dispersing into the area from untreated areas will probably cause recolonisation. In Kenya *S. neavei* has apparently been eradicated by the application of DDT to the relatively small streams in which this vector occurred, together with bush clearing.

In many areas ground application of larvicides is difficult, either because of the enormous size of the rivers requiring treatment or because breeding occurs in a large network of small streams and watercourses. Under these conditions aerial applications from small aircraft or helicopters have been used. Considerable information has been gained in North America on the chemical control of pestiferous blackflies. During the last 10 years much valuable experience has also been obtained in West Africa from the control of the vector, *S. damnosum*, under the auspices of the World Health Organization's 'Onchocerciasis Control Programme' (OCP). This programme is currently responsible for larviciding, with temephos (Abate), all breeding places of *S. damnosum* in the Volta River Basin, involving seven West African countries. Because, in some areas, two species of the *S. damnosum* complex have developed resistance to temephos, the microbial insecticide *Bacillus thuringiensis* var. *israelensis* is now used in these areas. This vast internationally backed control scheme started spraying operations in 1975 and will probably continue to do so for 20 years or more. If the vector population is reduced and held to a very low level then onchocerciasis transmission will be interrupted, but as the adult worms live in man for as long as 15 years control must be extended over this period to allow the disease to die out in the human population.

Chapter 5
Phlebotomine Sandflies

There are some 600 species of phlebotomine sandflies in five genera within the subfamily Phlebotominae of the family Psychodidae. Species in three genera, *Phlebotomus*, *Lutzomyia* and *Sergentomyia*, suck blood from vertebrates, the former two are the more important medically as they contain disease vectors. The genus *Phlebotomus* occurs only in the Old World, especially in southern parts of the northern temperate areas such as the Mediterranean region. The genus also occurs in the Old World tropics, but there are not many species in tropical Africa, especially West Africa. Most *Phlebotomus* species inhabit semi-arid and savanna areas in preference to forests. *Lutzomyia* species by contrast are found only in the New World tropics, occuring mostly in the forested areas of Central and South America.

Sergentomyia species are also confined to the Old World, being especially common in the Indian subregion, but also occurring in other areas such as Africa and Central Asia. A few species of *Sergentomyia* bite man, but they are not considered to be important in the transmission of disease to man.

Adult flies are often called sandflies. However, this can be confusing because in some parts of the world the small biting midges of the Ceratopogonidae (Chapter 6) and blackflies (Simuliidae, Chapter 4) are called sandflies. The most important species include *Phlebotomus papatasi*, *P. sergenti*, *P. major syriacus*, *P. argentipes*, *P. ariasi*, *P. perniciosus*, *Lutzomyia longipalpis* and species of the *Lutzomyia flaviscutellata* complex. In both the Old and New Worlds sandflies are vectors of leishmaniasis; the virus responsible for sandfly fever, and a parasite causing a disease called Bartonellosis (Carrión's disease).

EXTERNAL MORPHOLOGY

No details are given for distinguishing between the adults of *Phlebotomus*, *Lutzomyia* and *Sergentomyia* because this requires specialised knowledge and detailed examination; generally species biting man in the Old World will be *Phlebotomus* and in the New World *Lutzomyia*.

Adult phlebotomine sandflies can be readily recognised by their minute size (1·3–3·5 mm in length), hairy appearance, relatively large black eyes and their relatively long and stilt-like legs. The only other blood-sucking flies which are as small as this are some species of biting midges (Ceratopogonidae), but these have non-hairy wings and differ in many other details (Chapter 6). Phlebotomine sandflies have the head, thorax, wings and abdomen densely covered with long hairs. The antennae are long and composed of small bead-like segments with short hairs; they are similar in both sexes. The mouthparts, short and inconspicuous, are adapted for blood-sucking. At their base are a pair of five-segmented maxillary palps which are relatively conspicuous and droop downwards.

Wings are lanceolate in outline and quite distinct from the wings of other biting flies. The Phlebotominae can be distinguished from the very small, non-biting flies of the family of Psychodidae, which they superficially resemble, by the wings. In sandflies the wings are held erect over the body when the fly is at rest, whereas in non-biting psychodid flies they are folded, roof-like, over the body. The wing venation also differs. In phlebotomine sandflies, but not in the other subfamilies of Psychodidae, vein 2 branches twice, although this may not be apparent unless most of the hairs are rubbed from the wing veins (Fig. 5.1).

The abdomen is moderately long and in the female more or less rounded at the tip. In males it terminates in a prominent pair of claspers which give the end of the abdomen an upturned appearance.

Identification of adult phlebotomine sandflies to species is difficult and usually necessitates the examination of internal structures, such as the arrangement of the teeth on the cibarial armature, the shape of the spermatheca in females, and in males the structure of the external genitalia (terminalia).

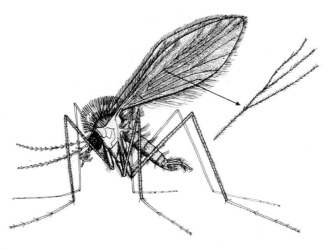

Fig. 5.1 Adult male phlebotomine sandfly, showing terminal abdominal claspers of the genitalia, and diagrammatic representation of double branching of wing vein 2.

LIFE-CYCLE

The minute eggs (0·3–0·4 mm) are more or less ovoid in shape and usually brown or black and careful examination under a microscope reveals that they are patterned, as shown in Fig. 5.2. Some 15–100 eggs are laid singly at each oviposition. They are deposited in small cracks and holes in the ground, at the base of termite mounds, in cracks in masonry, on stable floors, in poultry houses, amongst leaf litter and in between buttress roots of forest

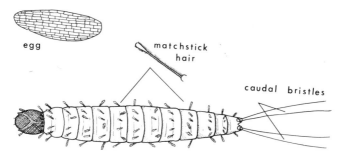

Fig. 5.2 Egg of phlebotomine sandfly showing mosaic-type pattern, and larva with matchstick hairs and caudal bristles.

trees, etc. The type of oviposition site varies greatly according to species.

Although eggs are not laid in water they require a moist microhabitat with a high humidity. They are unable to withstand desiccation and hatch after about 6–17 days under optimum conditions. However, hatching may be prolonged in cooler weather. Larvae are mainly scavengers, feeding on organic matter, such as fungi, decaying forest leaves, semi-rotting vegetation, animal faeces and decomposing bodies of arthropods. Although some species, especially of the genus *Phlebotomus*, occur in semi-arid areas, the actual larval habitats must have a high degree of humidity. Larvae can usually survive if their breeding places are temporarily flooded.

There are four larval instars. The mature larva is 3–6 mm long and has a well defined black head which is provided with a pair of small mandibles, the body is greyish or yellowish and 12-segmented (Fig. 5.2). The first seven abdominal segments have small pseudopods but the most striking feature of the larva is the presence, on the head and all body segments, of conspicuous thick bristles with feathered stems, and which in many species have slightly enlarged tips. They are called matchstick hairs and identify the larvae as those of phlebotomine sandflies. In most species the last abdominal segment bears two pairs of conspicuous long hairs called the caudal bristles. The first-instar larva has two single bristles not two pairs.

Larval development is completed after 19–60 days, the duration depending on species, temperature and availability of food. In temperate areas and arid regions species may overwinter as diapausing fully grown larvae. Prior to pupation the larva assumes an almost erect position in the habitat, the skin then splits open and the pupa wriggles out. The larval skin is not completely cast off but remains attached to the end of the pupa. The presence of this skin, with its characteristic two pairs of caudal bristles, aids in the recognition of phlebotomine pupae. The pupal shape is as shown in Fig. 5.3. Adults emerge from the pupae after about 7–14 days. The life-cycle, from oviposition to adult emergence, may be 28–100 days, depending on species and temperature; during cooler periods of the year the duration of the life-cycle may be extended. In temperate areas adults die off in late summer or autumn and the species overwinter as larvae, and the adults emerge the following spring.

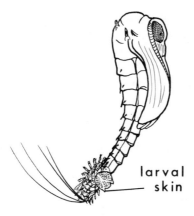

larval
skin

Fig. 5.3 Pupa of phlebotomine sandfly with larval skin still attached.

It is usually extremely difficult to find larvae or pupae of sandflies and relatively little is known about their biology and ecology.

Adult behaviour

Both sexes feed on plant juices and sugary secretions but females
in addition suck blood from a variety of vertebrates, including
livestock, dogs, urban and wild rodents, snakes, lizards and am-
phibians; a few species feed on birds. In the Old World many
Phlebotomus species bite man, whereas most species of *Sergentomyia* feed mainly on reptiles and rarely bite man. In the tropical
Americas *Lutzomyia* species feed on a variety of mammals including man. Biting is usually restricted to crepuscular and nocturnal
periods but man may be bitten during the day in darkened rooms,
or in forests during overcast days. Most species feed out of doors
(exophagic) but a few also feed indoors (endophagic). Adults are
weak fliers and do not usually disperse more than a few hundred
metres from their breeding places. Consequently biting may be
localised to a few areas. (Occasionally, however, such as in the
Crimea they have been reported flying up to 1200–1500 m.) Sandflies have a characteristic hopping type of flight so that there may
be several short flights and landings before females settle on their
hosts. Windy weather inhibits their flight activities and biting.
Because of their very short mouthparts they are unable to bite
through clothing.

During the day adult sandflies rest in sheltered, dark and humid sites, but on dry surfaces, such as on tree trunks, on ground litter and foliage of forest, in animal burrows, termite mounds, tree holes, rock fissures, caves, cracks in the ground and inside human and animal habitations. Species that commonly rest in houses (endophilic) before or after feeding on man are often referred to as domestic or peridomestic species. Examples are *Phlebotomus papatasi* in the Mediterranean area and *Lutzomyia longipalpis* in South America.

In temperate areas of the Old World sandflies are seasonal in their appearance and adults occur only in the summer months. In tropical areas some species appear to be common more or less throughout the year, but in other species there may be well marked changes in abundance of adults related to the dry and wet seasons.

MEDICAL IMPORTANCE

Annoyance

Apart from their importance as disease vectors, sandflies may constitute a serious, but usually localised, biting nuisance. In previously sensitised people their bites may result in severe and almost intolerable irritations, a condition known in the Middle East as Harara.

Leishmaniasis

This is a term used to describe a number of closely related diseases caused by several distinct species, subspecies and strains of *Leishmania* parasites. Phlebotomine sandflies are the only known vectors. Parasites are ingested by females with a blood-meal. They develop a flagellum with which they attach themselves to the gut wall, multiply within the insect's stomach and then migrate to the anterior part of the mid-gut and from there to the oesophagus. After about 4-12 days the infective forms are found in the mouthparts from where they are introduced into a new host during feeding. It appears that previous feeding by females on plant juices aids the survival of the parasite in the insect's gut.

Most types of leishmaniasis are zoonoses. The degree of involvement of man varies greatly from area to area. The epidemiology is complex and largely determined by the species, or even strains, of sandflies, their ecology and behaviour, the availability of a wide range of hosts and also by the species and strains of *Leishmania* parasites. In some areas, for example, sandflies will transmit the disease almost entirely amongst wild or domesticated animals, with little or no human involvement, whereas elsewhere animals may provide an important reservoir of infection for man. In India the disease may be transmitted between man by sandflies, with animals taking little, if any, part in its transmission.

Leishmaniasis occurs in two main forms, dermal (cutaneous) and visceral leishmaniasis. Old World dermal leishmaniasis (Oriental sore, cutaneous leishmaniasis) is caused by *Leishmania tropica*, and in Central Asia (mainly Russia) gerbils and ground squirrels are the principal animal reservoirs. In other areas, such as western India, the Middle East, Mediterranean countries and North Africa, dogs are important reservoirs but rodents may also be involved. Important vectors of dermal leishmaniasis include *Phlebotomus papatasi*, *P. caucasicus* and *P. sergenti*.

American dermal leishmaniasis (including mucocutaneous forms = espundia) is found from Mexico down to Argentina and is caused by several *Leishmania* species, such as the *Le. braziliensis* and *Le. mexicana* complexes, which normally infect a wide variety of forest rodents, marsupials, armadillos, edentates, primates, sloths and also domestic dogs. The disease is spread by several species of *Lutzomyia* including the *L. flaviscutellata* complex, *L. wellcomei*, *L. intermedia* and *L. umbratilis*.

The visceral form of *Leishmania* in the Old World (kala-azar) is cased by *Le. donovani* in most areas of its distribution, such as asiatic Russia, India, China, Kenya and Sudan, but by *Le. infantum* in the Mediterranean area through to the Central Asian area. In the Mediterranean region dogs and foxes are the most important reservoirs and the major vectors are *P. perniciosus*, *P. ariasis* and *P. major major*, while in China dogs are also reservoirs and the important vector is *P. chinensis*. In India neither dogs nor any other animal appears to act as a reservoir and the disease is transmitted to man mainly by *P. argentipes*. In the Middle East *P. major syriacus* is a vector and wild and domestic dogs appear to be the most important reservoirs.

In South America both wild and domesticated dogs are reservoirs of the visceral form and the vector is usually *L. longipalpis*.

Bartonellosis

This disease is sometimes called Oroya fever or Carrión's disease and is encountered in arid mountainous areas of the Andes in Peru, Ecuador and Colombia. It is caused by a small rod-like micro-organism named *Bartonella bacilliformis* and is transmitted by *L. verrucarum* and possibly by other *Lutzomyia* species. Transmission is probably entirely by contamination of the mouthparts.

Sandfly fever

Sometimes called papataci fever or 3-day fever, this disease is caused by more than 27 strains of a virus transmitted primarily by *P. papatasi*. Females become infective 6–10 days after taking an infected blood-meal. It appears that the infected females can lay eggs containing the virus and that these can eventually give rise to infected adults. This is an example of transovarial transmission, a phenomenon that is more common in the transmission of various tick-borne diseases (Chapter 17). Sandfly fever occurs mainly in the Mediterranean region but extends up the Nile and also into India, Pakistan and probably China where, in the absence of *P. papatasi* other *Phlebotomus* species are likely involved in its transmission.

CONTROL

Leishmaniasis has not in the past been considered a sufficiently important disease to justify expenditure on controlling the insect vectors. Phlebotomine sandflies, are, however, very susceptible to most insecticides: the only case of resistance is to DDT in India. In nearly all areas where residual insecticides, particularly DDT, have been used to control the *Anopheles* vectors of malaria there have been drastic reductions of sandfly populations followed by interruption of leishmaniasis transmission. With the cessation of spraying, sandflies usually return, and transmission is renewed.

Dosages of 1 or $2 \mathrm{g\,m^{-2}}$ of DDT or $0.4 \mathrm{g\,m^{-2}}$ of HCH, applied as a residual house-spray have given excellent control of *Phlebotomus* species. It seems probable that insecticidal fogging of the outdoor resting sites of adults should give good, although most likely temporary, control.

Personal protection can be achieved by the use of efficient insect repellents, such as diethyltoluamide, dimethylphthalate or trimethyl pentanediol, or the use of very fine screens or sandfly nets. A disadvantage of using screens and nets with very small holes, is that they reduce ventilation causing it to be unpleasantly hot in screened houses or under sandfly nets over beds.

Chapter 6
Biting Midges

Biting midges belong to the family Ceratopogonidae, which has over 60 genera. Midges have a more or less world-wide distribution, the most widely distributed genus being *Culicoides* which is found in both tropical and subarctic areas. Only *Lasiohelea* and the genera *Leptoconops*, and most importantly *Culicoides*, of which over 1000 species have been described, feed on vertebrates including man, and therefore are of considerable medical importance. In many parts of the world species of *Culicoides*, and in the Americas also *Leptoconops*, can constitute a serious biting problem. *Culicoides milnei* and *C. grahamii* are vectors of *Dipetalonema perstans*, and *C. grahamii* and possibly *C. milnei* are vectors of *D. streptocerca*. *C. furens* is a vector of *Mansonella ozzardi*. These filarial parasites are usually regarded as non-pathogenic to man.

EXTERNAL MORPHOLOGY

A generalised description is given of the adults of *Culicoides*.

Adult *Culicoides* are sometimes known as midges or biting midges and, especially in the Americas, as 'no-see-ums' or 'punkies', and in Australia and other countries as sandflies. This latter name is unfortunate and should be avoided because phlebotomines (Chapter 5) and occasionally simuliids (Chapter 4) may also be referred to as sandflies. The most appropriate common name is biting midges; this terminology serves to distinguish them from other small non-biting flies which are often referred to as midges.

Adults are very small insects being only about 1·5 mm long and with the phlebotomines constitute the smallest biting flies attacking man.

The small head bears a prominent pair of eyes and a pair of relatively long antennae. As in mosquitoes, males do not take blood-meals and have feathery or plumose antennae whereas the

blood-sucking females have non-plumose antennae. The biting
mouthparts are very small and inconspicuous and they do not
project forwards but hang down vertically from the head. The
arrangement and structure of the mouthparts are very similar to
those of simuliids (Chapter 4). In many species the thorax is
covered dorsally with very small but distinct black spots and
markings. In addition to these dark markings, a pair of black,
small but elongated, depressions, known as the humeral pits, are
present in all *Culicoides* species on the dorsal surface of the
anterior part of the thorax. The presence of these pits distinguishes the genus *Culicoides* from *Lasiohelea* and *Leptoconops*.
The wings are short and relatively broad, and apart from the first
veins their venation is faint. The wings lack scales but in many
species are covered with minute hairs—these are seen only under
a dissecting microscope. In most *Culicoides* species the wings have
contrasting dark and milky white spots or patches (Fig. 6.1). In
life the wings are placed over the abdomen like the blades of a
closed pair of scissors (Fig. 6.1). The legs are relatively short.

The abdomen is dull grey, yellowish brown or blackish and in
the female is more or less rounded at its tip, in the male there is
a pair of small, but conspicuous, claspers.

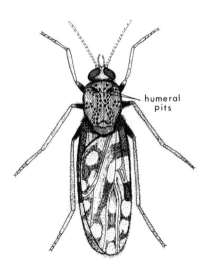

Fig. 6.1 Adult *Culicoides* showing patterned wing and thoracic humeral pits.

LIFE-CYCLE

The eggs are dark, cylindrical or curved and banana-shaped, and are about 0·5 mm long (Fig. 6.2c). They are laid in batches of about 30–250 on the surface of mud, wet soil, especially that near swamps and marshes including salt water marshes, on decaying leaf litter, humus, manure, or on plants and other objects near or partially submerged in water, in tree holes, in semi-rotting vegetation and in the cut stumps of banana plants (for example *Culicoides milnei* and *C. grahamii*). The type of oviposition site selected depends on the species.

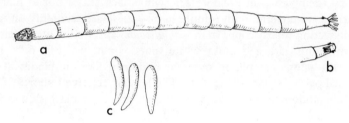

Fig. 6.2 (a) Larvae of *Culicoides* with two four-lobed retractile papillae extending from last abdominal segment; (b) last abdominal segment with papillae retracted inside; (c) *Culicoides* eggs.

Eggs usually hatch within about 2–9 days, depending on temperature and species, some temperate species overwinter as eggs. There are four larval instars and the fully grown larva is cylindrical, whitish and about 5–6 mm long. It has a small, dark, conical-shaped head followed by 11 body segments. The last segment terminates in two four-lobed retractile papillae (Fig. 6.2a). These are not always readily seen in preserved larvae because they are often retracted within the last abdominal segment (Fig. 6.2b). *Culicoides* larvae are best recognised by the combination of a small dark head followed by a segmented body devoid of any obvious structures, and when they are extruded, by the presence of terminal papillae. When alive they can also be recognised by their serpentine swimming motions.

Larvae feed mainly on decaying vegetable matter and occur in many different types of habitats, including fresh or salt water marshes and swamps, edges of ponds, boggy and semi-waterlogged areas, and in specialised habitats such as horse and cow excreta, tree holes and rotting cacti. When the water level in swamps and marshes rises the larvae of many species migrate to the damp soil and mud at the edges to avoid becoming completely submerged. Some important pest species breed in sandy areas near the seashore. Larvae are difficult to find and are rarely encountered unless special surveys are made to collect them.

In warm countries larval development is completed within 14–25 days, but in temperate regions many species overwinter and remain as larvae for 7 months or more. Species occupying marshy habitats frequently migrate to the drier peripheral areas for pupation. However, in species that are aquatic the pupae float at the water surface.

The pupa (Fig. 6.3) is 2–4 mm long and readily recognised by the following combination of characters: (i) a pair of breathing trumpets on the cephalothorax which appear to be composed of two segments; (ii) abdominal segments bearing small but conspicuous tubercles ending in a fine hair; and (iii) a prominent pair of horn-like processes on the last abdominal segment. The pupal period lasts 3–10 days.

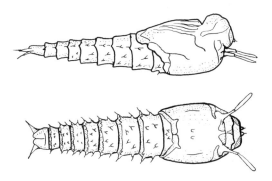

Fig. 6.3 Lateral and dorsal views of a *Culicoides* pupa.

Adult behaviour

Adults of both sexes feed on naturally occurring sugar solutions. In addition females take blood-meals from man and a variety of mammals and birds. Adults bite at any time of the day and night, but many species are particularly active and troublesome in the evenings and first half of the night. In contrast *C. grahamii* bites mainly in the early part of the mornings. Because of their short mouthparts, biting midges are not as successful in biting through clothing as are mosquitoes, tabanids and tsetse flies, all of which have a longer proboscis. For this reason midges often appear in swarms or clouds around the head, biting the face, especially the forehead and scalp. They also bite other exposed parts such as the hands and arms, and the legs of people wearing shorts. Most species bite only outdoors, but a few including *C. milnei* and *C. grahamii* will enter houses to feed on man (endophagic). Adults normally fly only a few hundred metres from their larval habitats, but they may be dispersed considerably further by wind.

MEDICAL IMPORTANCE

Annoyance

Biting midges are very small, but what they lack in size they can make up for in numbers—as has been said, one midge is an entomological curiosity, a thousand sheer hell! In several areas of the world, as dissimilar as the west coast of Scotland, the Caribbean and the sunny regions of California and Florida, biting midges can be a serious ecomonic threat to the tourist industry. The persistent biting of large numbers of midges can make out of door recreational activities impossible, not only at dusk but often during much of the day. In some areas they have even prevented the continuation of harvesting and other out of door work during the evenings.

Important pest species in southern areas of North America down to Brazil include *C. furens* which breeds in salt marshes and other saline coastal habitats. In North America *Leptoconops torrens* and *L. becquaerti*, which also breed in sandy soils and coastal areas, can be serious pests. In Europe *C. impunctatus* and many other species are troublesome biters, while in Madagascar, the Seychelles and Brunei *L. spinosifrons* can cause a considerable biting problem.

Filarial infections

A few *Culicoides* species are vectors of parasites to man. In Africa, especially West and Central, but also in parts of East Africa as far south as Zimbabwe, *Dipetalonema* (=*Acanthocheilonema*) *perstans* is transmitted to man by *Culicoides milnei* (=*austeni*), and possibly by *C. grahamii*. *Dipetalonema perstans* also occurs in Trinidad and South America where it is transmitted by other *Culicoides* species. In the rain forests of Ghana, Burkina Faso, Nigeria, Cameroon and Zaire, *Dipetalonema* (=*A.*) *streptocerca* is transmitted by *C. grahamii*, and possibly *C. milnei*. These species breed in the rotting, cut stumps of banana and plantain plants.

In Mexico, Panama, the West Indies and South America *Mansonella ozzardi* is transmitted by *Culicoides* species, mainly *C. furens*, but other species such as *C. phlebotomus* are also likely to be involved. (See Chapter 4 regarding the role of simuliids in the transmission of this filarial parasite.)

Microfilariae of all these parasites are non-periodic, they are ingested with a blood-meal and pass through a similar developmental cycle to other filarial parasites in mosquitoes. That is, they undergo morphological changes, invade the thoracic flight muscles, moult twice and then migrate to the head and after about 9–12 days pass down the proboscis. The infective 3rd-stage larvae are deposited on the skin of the host when the female takes a blood-meal. The salivary glands of *Culicoides* play no part in the transmission of these parasites. None of the three filarial parasites carried by midges appears to cause much harm to man, they are usually regarded as non-pathogenic, although morbidity or allergic reactions may sometimes occur. In general the Ceratopogonidae are not considered as very important vectors of disease to man.

CONTROL

Because many of the major pest species breed in extensive and often diffuse habitats, such as fresh and salt water marshes and wet coastal sands, whose limits are usually difficult to define, it is usually very difficult to reduce larval breeding substantially. For effective control often large areas of land or marsh must be drained or sprayed with insecticides.

Although larval habitats can be eradicated by draining or filling this is often costly, laborious and in many areas impractical. Sometimes semi-aquatic sites, such as muddy or marshy areas, can be impounded and flooded under 5–8 cm of water to ensure that the soil is never exposed, thus destroying suitable habitats. This type of environmental control can be effective against some species but be ineffective against others. If maintained such methods have the advantage of giving permanent control. However, although they avoid contaminating the environment with insecticides they in themselves result in completely changing the habitat.

Insecticidal applications can sometimes be effective. The best and most lasting control is usually obtained by spraying breeding sites with organochlorine insecticides, but heavy rainfall is needed to wash the insecticides through the surface vegetation to the underlying soil and mud harbouring the midge larvae. Dieldrin, at rates of about $1-4\,kg\,ha^{-1}$, has given good control against *Culicoides* and *Leptoconops* species in the USA where diazinon, at about $2\,kg\,ha^{-1}$, has also been successfully employed against *Leptoconops* species; chlorphyrifos (Dursban), another organophosphate insecticide, has also proved useful in midge control.

Thermal insecticidal aerosols or ultra-low-volume (ULV) applications have sometimes been used to kill adults resting in vegetation, but the effects are very short-lived and sprayed areas are soon invaded by midges flying in from unsprayed areas.

Limited personal protection can be achieved by the use of suitable repellents such as diethyltoluamide, dimethylphthalate or trimethyl pentanediol. Mosquito nets and screening used to keep out houseflies and mosquitoes may not exclude the much smaller biting midges. To prevent them from passing through protective nets and screens a very small mesh size must be used, but a disadvantage is that this substantially reduces air flow and ventilation. Nets and screens can be treated with insecticides such as 6 per cent malathion or propoxur (Baygon) or with synthetic pyrethroids like permethrin. Such treated nets may remain effective for several months, after which they can be re-impregnated.

Chapter 7
Horseflies

Horseflies, clegs and other large biting flies belong to the family
Tabanidae, which comprises many genera and over 3000 species.
The most important from the medical point of view are certain
species of *Chrysops*, *Tabanus* and *Haematopota*. *Chrysops*, mainly
C. silacea and *C. dimidiata*, are vectors in West and Central Africa
of *Loa loa*. In the USA *C. discalis* is a vector of tularaemia,
caused by *Pasteurella tularensis*. Tabanidae possibly play a very
minor role in the mechanical spread of human and animal trypanosomiasis. In Central and South America tabanids are involved
in the transmission of a form of *Trypanosoma vivax* to cattle and
sheep.

The Tabanidae have a world-wide distribution. Species of *Tabanus* and *Chrysops* are found in temperate and tropical areas, but
Haematopota is absent from South America and Australia and is
uncommon in North America.

EXTERNAL MORPHOLOGY

A generalised description is presented of the Tabanidae, with
special reference to the genera *Chrysops*, *Tabanus* and *Haematopota*.

Tabanids are medium to very large flies (5-25 mm). Many,
especially of the genus *Tabanus*, are robust and heavily built, and
this genus contains the largest biting flies, some attaining a wing
span of 6·5 cm. The colouration of tabanids varies from very dark
brown or black to lighter reddish-brown, yellow or greenish; frequently the abdomen and thorax have stripes or patches of contrasting colours (Fig. 7.1). The head is large and, viewed from
above, is more or less semicircular in outline (Fig. 7.2), it is often
described as semi-lunar. The head bears a conspicuous pair of
compound eyes which in life may be marked with contrasting
iridescent colours, such as greens and reds or even purplish hues,

115

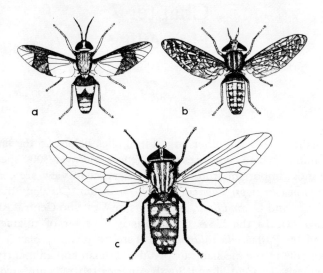

Fig. 7.1 Adult Tabanidae. (a) *Chrysops*; (b) *Haematopota*; (c) *Tabanus*.

arranged in bands, zig-zags or spots. Adults can be sexed by examination of their eyes. In the female there is a distinct space on top of the head between the eyes; this is known as a dichoptic condition (Fig. 7.2). In females of some species this space between the eyes may be narrow, while in others, especially *Chrysops*, it is quite large. In the males the eyes are so large that they occupy

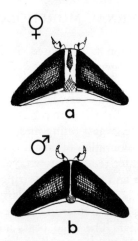

Fig. 7.2 Dorsal view of tabanid heads. (a) female with dichoptic eyes; (b) male with holoptic eyes.

almost all of the head and either touch each other on top of the head or are very narrowly separated, this being known as a holoptic condition (Fig. 7.2).

The antennae are relatively small but stout. They consist of three segments; the last is subdivided into three or four small divisions by annulations. Unlike the Muscidae, Glossinidae and Calliphoridae there is no antennal arista. The size and shape of the antennae serve to distinguish the genera *Chrysops*, *Haematopota* and *Tabanus* (Fig. 7.3). The mouthparts of female Tabanidae

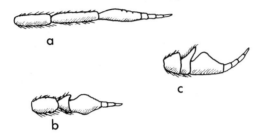

Fig. 7.3 Antennae of adult tabanids. (a) *Chrysops*; (b) *Haematopota*; (c) *Tabanus*.

are stout and adapted for biting and, unlike those of tsetse flies, mosquitoes and *Stomoxys*, they do not project forwards but point downwards from the head. Only female tabanids take blood-meals.

The thorax is stout and bears a pair of wings which have two submarginal and five posterior cells and a completely closed discal cell in approximately the centre of the wing (Fig. 7.4). Although the wing venation alone may not be sufficient to identify the Tabanidae from all other Diptera, it nevertheless serves as a useful guide when considered with other characters, such as the

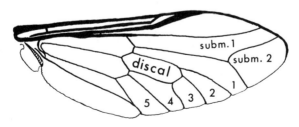

Fig. 7.4 Wing of adult tabanid, showing discal cell, two submarginal cells and five posterior cells.

shape and structure of the antennae and biting mouthparts. The wings may be completely clear and devoid of colour or have areas of brown colouration, or they may be distinctly banded, or appear mottled or speckled due to the presence of greyish patches (see Fig. 7.1). When adults are at rest the wings are placed either like a pair of open scissors over the abdomen or at a roof-like angle completely obscuring the abdomen. The presence or absence of coloured areas on the wings and the way in which they are held over the body provides useful additional characters for distinguishing between *Chrysops*, *Tabanus* and *Haematopota* (see pp. 121–2).

The abdomen is usually broad and stout, and in unfed flies characteristically flattened dorsoventrally. It may be a more or less uniform dark brown, blackish, light brown, reddish-brown, yellowish or even greenish, or alternatively marked with contrasting coloured stripes or patches.

LIFE-CYCLE

Males feed only on naturally occurring sugary secretions. Females also feed on sugary substances but in addition they bite a wide variety of mammals such as domestic animals, especially horses and cattle, deer and many other herbivores, carnivores, monkeys, reptiles, amphibia. A few species even attack birds. They also feed on man.

Some 100–1000 eggs, the number depending on the species, are deposited by female tabanids on the underside of objects such as leaves, grassy vegetation, plant stems, twigs, small branches, stones and rocks. These oviposition sites overhang, or are adjacent to, the larval habitats, which are mainly muddy, aquatic or semi-aquatic sites (see p. 119). The eggs, which are firmly glued to the substrate in an upright position, are covered with a coating that is impervious to water, i.e. they are waterproofed. They are usually arranged in more or less lozenge-shaped patterns (Fig. 7.5a) and are mostly creamy white, greyish or blackish. They measure 1–2·5 mm in length and are curved or approximately cigar-shaped. They hatch after about 4–14 days, the time depending on both temperature and species. After wriggling out of the eggs the young larvae drop down on to the underlying mud or water.

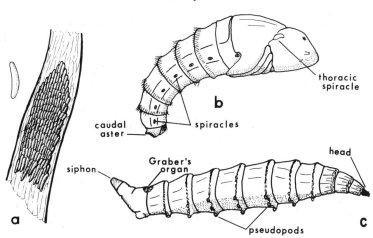

Fig. 7.5 Immature stages of tabanids. (a) single egg and egg mass glued to a piece of grass; (b) a pupa; (c) a larva.

Larvae are cylindrical and rather pointed at both ends (Fig. 7.5c). They are creamy white, brown or even greenish and have a very small black head which can be retracted into the thorax. There are 11 well differentiated body segments. Larvae are readily recognised by the prominent raised tyre-like rings which encircle most body segments. Segments 4–10, but not the last, have one pair of lateral and two pairs of ventral (a total of six) conspicuous roundish protuberances called pseudopods. The presence of the prominent rings and these pseudopods readily identify larvae of tabanids. The last abdominal segment bears a short siphon dorsally which can be retracted into the abdomen, and a pyriform structure known as Graber's organ which is composed of 15 or less black globular bodies. This can be readily seen with the aid of a hand lens or microscope and is unique to tabanid larvae. This organ is well provided with nerves and seems to be sensory, but its exact function is not clearly understood.

Larvae live in mud, rotting vegetation, humus, damp soil, in shallow and often muddy water, at the edges of small pools, swamps, ditches or slowly flowing streams. In aquatic habitats larvae sometimes adhere to floating leaves, logs, or other debris. A few species breed in tree holes. Some species occur in brackish habitats, while larvae of certain *Tabanus* and *Haematopota* species are found in the relatively dry soils of pastures and in the earth near the bases of trees. Larvae breathe atmospheric oxygen through the short siphon at the posterior end of the body, and because they are poor swimmers aquatic species are usually found only in shallow waters. They move rather sluggishly in their muddy, aquatic or semi-aquatic environment. In some species, in particular *Chrysops*, the larvae are scavengers, feeding on detritus and a variety of dead and decaying vegetable and animal matter; while larvae of *Tabanus* and *Haematopota* are predacious or cannibalistic.

Larval development is prolonged. In both temperate and tropical countries many species spend 1–2 years as larvae, and several temperate species may remain as larvae for as long as 3 years. Larvae, however, are not easily found and relatively little is known about the life-cycle of many species, but there appear to be 4–11 larval instars. Depending upon the species mature larvae may be 1–6 cm long. Prior to pupation mature larvae migrate to drier areas at the periphery of the larval habitat where they pupate. The pupa is partially buried in the mud or soil in an upright position and, superficially, looks like a chrysalis of a butterfly (Fig. 7.5b). It is 7–40 mm long, size depending on the species, distinctly curved and is usually brown. The head and thorax are combined to form a distinct cephalothorax which has a pair of lateral and relatively large, ear-shaped spiracles. The abdomen is composed of eight well defined segments, the first seven are supplied with a pair of lateral spiracles, while segments 2–6 have an encircling row of small backwardly directed spines. A few spines are also present ventrally on segment 7. The short terminal eighth abdominal segment is provided with six lobes which bear spine-like processes, known collectively as the caudal aster. The pupal period lasts about 5–20 days.

Adult behaviour

Females of most species feed during the daylight hours and are especially active in bright sunshine. They locate their prey mainly by sight, but a few species feed at night. Tabanids are powerful fliers and may disperse many kilometres.

Most tabanids inhabit woods and forests. Many *Chrysops* species are common in low-lying marshy scrub areas or swampy woods; some species, however, are found in more open savanna and grassland areas. Adults do not usually enter houses to feed, but *C. silacea* is an exception. Other species may be found in houses, especially on windows, but often these have entered accidentally and are trying to escape.

Because of their large and rather broad mouthparts, bites from tabanids are deep and painful, sometimes especially so, and wounds inflicted by tabanids frequently continue to bleed after the female has departed. Due to their painful bites they are frequently disturbed when feeding on either man or other hosts. As a result several small blood-meals may be taken from the same or different hosts before the female has obtained a complete meal. This interrupted feeding behaviour increases their likelihood of being mechanical vectors of disease. Because of their preference for dark objects they often prefer to bite through coloured clothing when attacking Caucasians rather than exposed areas of pale skin, in this respect they behave like tsetse flies.

In both temperate and tropical areas the occurrence of adults is seasonal. In temperate countries adults usually die off at the end of the summer and a new population emerges in the spring or summer of the following year. In the tropics the flies may not completely disappear in the dry months. However, their numbers are normally much reduced. Maximum numbers of biting flies usually appear towards the beginning of the rainy season.

Identification of adult *Chrysops*, *Tabanus* and *Haematopota*

Chrysops *species (deerflies, green heads, mangrove flies)*

These are medium sized flies ranging in size from that of a housefly to a tsetse fly. In life most species have iridescent eyes, commonly with spots of red, green or purple. The wings, which are held partially over the abdomen in an open scissor-like fashion, usually have one or more transverse bands of brownish colour (see Fig. 7.1a). In many species the abdomen is blackish with orange or yellow patches or bands.

The most reliable method of distinguishing *Chrysops* species from *Tabanus* and *Haematopota* is by the antennae. In *Chrysops* these are long; the second segment is neither short nor bears a projection (see Fig. 7.3a), while the third segment has four small subdivisions. The hind tibiae have apical spurs; these are absent from *Tabanus* and *Haematopota*.

Chrysops has a world-wide distribution.

Tabanus *species* (*horseflies*)

Medium to very large flies. The eyes are frequently brownish but may be iridescent, the markings are usually in the form of horizontal bands. The wings, which are held over the body much as in *Chrysops*, are often clear (see Fig. 7.1c), but in some species there are dark markings.

Tabanus species are readily identified by the shape and size of the antennae. Both the second and third antennal segments have small, but distinct projections on the upper surface (see Fig. 7.3c), the third segment has four small subdivisions and is usually distinctly curved upwards. The antennae are much shorter than those of *Chrysops* species, and are therefore less conspicuous.

Tabanus has a world-wide distribution.

Haematopota (*clegs or stouts*)

Medium sized dark grey flies which are easily distinguished from *Tabanus* and *Chrysops* by the fact that in life the wings are folded roof-like over the abdomen. Moreover, in nearly all species the wings are dusty grey and speckled or mottled (see Fig. 7.1b). The eyes have zig-zag bands of iridescent colours. The antennae are similar to those of *Tabanus*, but usually longer. The third segment is straight, not curved as in *Tabanus*, has only three, not four, small subdivisions and does not bear a dorsal projection (see Fig. 7.3).

Haematopota species are not found in South America or Australia, and only very few species occur in North America. They are common in Europe, Asia, Africa, India and the Far East.

MEDICAL IMPORTANCE

Because females tend to be intermittent feeders, and are often disturbed during feeding, tabanids are particularly liable to be mechanical vectors. In this way they can spread anthrax and anaplasmosis, both of which can infect man. They are also mechanical vectors of *Trypanosoma evansi*, which causes a disease called Surra in camels, horses and dogs, often with fatal results; it does not infect man. In Central and South America tabanids are also mechanical vectors of *Trypanosoma vivax viennei* to livestock. This form of *vivax* does not infect man.

Because of their painful bites, tabanids may sometimes constitute a pest nuisance and make outdoor activities, whether recreational or work, difficult. Some people develop severe allergic
symptoms due to the large amount of saliva that is pumped into
the wound to prevent blood clotting.

Two diseases are spread to man by the Tabanidae. The less
important one is tularaemia (*Pasteurella tularensis*) which is
spread mechanically from horses, rabbits and other rodents. In
North America *C. discalis* is a vector, but other tabanids may also
transmit. The disease is also commonly spread by handling infected rodents, by ixodid tick bites and by eating insufficiently
cooked food.

Loiasis

The only important disease transmitted to man by tabanids is
loiasis, caused by the parasitic nematode *Loa loa* which undergoes
a developmental cycle in the fly. This disease occurs principally
in the equatorial rain forests of Sierra Leone westwards to Ghana
and then from Nigeria across Central Africa, the southern Sudan
and into western parts of Uganda. Diurnal periodic microfilariae
are found in the peripheral blood of man and are ingested by
tabanids with their blood-meal. In *Chrysops* species, in particular
C. silacea and *C. dimidiata*, many, but not all, the microfilariae
survive the process of blood digestion, penetrate the gut wall and
migrate to the abdominal and thoracic fat bodies. Here they grow,
moult twice and develop into shorter and fatter larval forms
(2 mm long), which, after 10–12 days, are able to migrate down
the proboscis. Infective larvae may be quite numerous in the fly
and are commonly found in the abdomen and thorax as well as in
the head and proboscis. When *Chrysops* feed on man the infective
worms migrate from other parts of the body to the proboscis and
enter the skin. They eventually develop into adult worms which
live in the subcutaneous tissues of man. Microfilariae of *Loa loa*
are more or less absent from the blood circulation of man at night
but appear in it during the day, especially in the morning, and
are therefore readily picked up by *C. silacea* and *C. dimidiata*
species which bite during the day. In Central Africa the vector
appears to be *C. distinctipennis*.

A similar parasite, which was previously considered to be *Loa
loa*, but which now appears to be a different, but closely related,

subspecies or strain (*Loa loa papionis*), occurs in some forest monkeys. The microfilariae appear in the peripheral blood at night and are picked up by *C. centurionis* and *C. langi*, species which are mainly crepuscular and nocturnal in their biting habits.

CONTROL

There are very few practical control measures to combat tabanids. In theory efficient drainage to remove not only standing water but to dry out marshy and muddy areas might reduce the numbers of species breeding in these habitats, but the cost of both locating the larval habitats, and carrying out drainage obviates this approach. Similarly, because of the difficulty of locating breeding places and their diffuse and large size, it is usually impossible to achieve control by the application of insecticides. Moreover, because the larvae of many species live below the surface of the ground, heavy dosage rates are needed for the insecticide to penetrate through the surface soil and vegetation to reach the larvae; these problems are somewhat similar to those encountered in the control of ceratopogonid larvae (Chapter 6).

Chapter 8
Tsetse Flies

There are 30 named species and subspecies of tsetse flies, all of which belong to the genus *Glossina*. Tsetse flies are restricted to tropical Africa from between, approximately, latitudes 15° north and 20° south, but extending to about 30° south along the eastern coastal area. Some species such as *G. morsitans* are found across West Africa to Central and East Africa, whereas others are more restricted in their distribution. For example, *G. palpalis* occurs only in the West African subregion.

Tsetse flies are vectors of both human and animal African trypanosomiasis, the disease in man being referred to as sleeping sickness. The most important species are *G. palpalis*, *G. tachinoides*, *G. fuscipes*, *G. pallidipes*, *G. swynnertoni* and *G. morsitans*.

EXTERNAL MORPHOLOGY

A general description of tsetse flies, without special reference to any particular species, is as follows. Adults are yellowish or brown-black robust flies that are rather larger (6–15 mm) than house-flies. In some species the abdominal segments are uniformly coloured while in others there may be lighter coloured transverse stripes and a median longitudinal one. Tsetse flies are readily distinguished from all other biting flies and similar sized non-biting flies by the combination of a rigid and forwardly projecting proboscis and a characteristic wing venation. In between veins 4 and 5 there is a closed cell which, with a little imagination, looks like an upside down hatchet (i.e. axe, cleaver or chopper), and is consequently often termed the hatchet cell (Figs. 8.1 and 8.2a). This one character serves to identify a fly as a tsetse. Tsetse flies also differ from most flies in that at rest the wings are placed over the abdomen like the closed blades of a pair of scissors (Fig. 8.1a).

A long pair of palps arise dorsally, very close to the proboscis and lie alongside it. They are difficult to distinguish except when

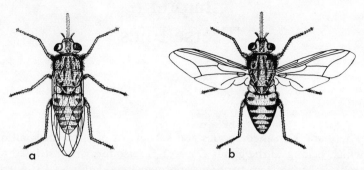

Fig. 8.1 Tsetse fly. (a) Wings folded over body like a pair of closed scissors; (b) wings pulled away to display abdomen and wing venation.

the tsetse fly is feeding and the proboscis is swung downwards while the palps remain projecting forwards (Fig. 8.2b). The first two antennal segments are small and inconspicuous but the third is relatively large and cylindrical and is also somewhat banana-shaped. This has near its base the arista which has branched

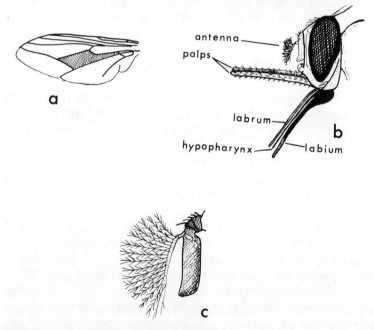

Fig. 8.2 Adult tsetse fly. (a) Wing showing shaded hatchet cell; (b) lateral view of head showing mouthparts, antenna and palps; (c) antenna showing plumose branching of hairs on arista.

hairs, but only on the upper surface, giving it a feathery appearance (Fig. 8.2c).

The proboscis is relatively large and has a bulbous base. When a tsetse feeds saliva containing anticoagulants is pumped down into the wound formed by the fly.

The dorsal surface of the thorax of a tsetse fly has a pattern of dark brown stripes and patches. The abdominal segments may be uniformly dark brown or blackish, or have transverse stripes and a median one of a lighter brown or yellowish colour. Although, as far as disease transmission is concerned, it may not be important to distinguish between the sexes because both take blood-meals, this can easily be done by examining the tip of the ventral surface of the abdomen. In the male tsetse fly there is a prominent raised, almost circular, knob-like structure called the hypopygium, which when unfolded reveals a pair of claspers. In the female there is no such knob-like protuberance.

Alimentary canal of the adult fly (Fig. 8.3)

A knowledge of the morphology of the alimentary canal and associated salivary glands is essential for an understanding of the life-cycle of trypanosomes within the tsetse.

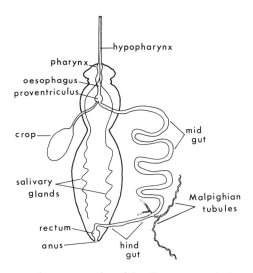

Fig. 8.3 Diagrammatic representation of the alimentary canal of a tsetse fly, and the thread-like salivary glands.

The food channel, formed by the apposition of the labrum and labium, leads to the pharynx and then to the oesophagus which has a slender duct leading to an oesophageal diverticulum, commonly called the crop. Just behind the oesophagus there is an important bulbous structure termed the proventriculus. The distal end of the proventriculus marks the end of the fore gut and beginning of the mid gut which in the tsetse fly is very long and convoluted. A peritrophic membrane, which plays an important part in the cyclical development of sleeping sickness trypanosomes (*Trypanosoma brucei gambiense*, *T. brucei rhodesiense*) in the tsetse fly, is secreted by the epithelial cells in the anterior part of the proventriculus. The peritrophic membrane when first produced by the proventriculus is a very delicate, soft and almost fluid structure but as it passes back into the gut it hardens to form a thin but relatively tough sleeve, something like a sausage skin. This tube-like peritrophic membrane lines the entire length of the mid gut.

The junction of the four Malpighian tubules separates the mid gut from the hind gut, which terminates in a small dilated rectum and opens to the exterior through the anus.

The slender paired salivary glands originating in the head of the tsetse are enormously long, very convoluted and stretch back to almost the end of the abdomen. Anteriorly, the ducts from both glands unite in the head to form the common salivary duct which passes down the length of the hypopharynx.

LIFE-CYCLE

Feeding and reproduction

Both male and female tsetse flies bite man, a large variety of domesticated and wild mammals, and also reptiles and birds. No species of tsetse feeds exclusively on one type of host but most species show definite host preferences. For example, in East Africa *Glossina swynnertoni* feeds mainly on wild pigs and *G. morsitans* on wild and domesticated bovids and wild pigs, but in West Africa *G. morsitans* feeds mainly on warthogs. In East Africa *G. pallidipes* feeds principally on wild bovids, while in West Africa *G. palpalis* feeds predominantly on reptiles and man and *G. tachinoides* feeds on man and bovids, but in southern Nigeria predominantly on domestic pigs. They take blood-meals about every 2–3 days, although this interval may be reduced in dry, hot weather or prolonged for about 10 days in cool, humid conditions. Feeding is restricted to daylight hours and vision plays an important part in host location, dark moving objects being particularly attractive. On pale-skinned people, such as Caucasians, tsetse flies often prefer to bite through dark clothing such as socks, trousers and shorts in preference to settling on the skin. During feeding blood is sucked up the proboscis, passes to the crop and later to the stomach where digestion proceeds.

The different types of flies so far described in this book lay eggs—in marked contrast tsetse flies do not, instead they deposit larvae one at a time. (Adults of *Sarcophaga* and *Wohlfahrtia* also deposit larvae not eggs, see Chapter 10.)

After a female tsetse fly has been inseminated by a male and after it has taken a blood-meal, a single egg in one of the two ovaries completes maturation. It then passes down the common oviduct into the uterus where it is fertilised by the release of spermatozoa from the spermathecae. The egg hatches within the uterus after about 3–4 days, and the empty egg shell passes out through the genital orifice (vagina). The uterus is supplied with a conspicuous pair of branched secretory accessory glands which in tsetse flies are called the milk glands (Fig. 8.4). Fatty, nutrient fluid from these glands flows through a small duct to enter the

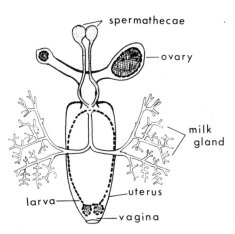

Fig. 8.4 Diagrammatic representation of the female reproductive system of a tsetse fly, with a full grown larva in the uterus.

uterus at its anterior end. The larva is orientated within the uterus so that its mouth is near the opening of the common duct of the milk glands. The secretions from these glands provide the larva with all the food it needs for growth and development. The larva passes through three instars in the female. Regular blood-meals must be taken by the female for a continuous and adequate provision of nutrient fluid from the milk glands. If the fly is unable to feed, the larva may fail to complete its development and as a consequence be 'aborted'.

Larval development is completed after about 4–5 days, by which time the 3rd and final instar larva is 8–9 mm long. It is creamy white in colour and composed of 12 visible segments, the last of which bears a pair of prominent dark protuberances called the polypneustic lobes (Fig. 8.5b), which are respiratory structures. A female containing a fully developed larva is easily recognised because the fly's abdomen is enlarged and stretched, i.e. the fly is obviously 'pregnant'. Furthermore, the black polypneustic lobes can be seen through her abdominal integument.

The mature 3rd-instar larva wriggles out, posterior end first, from the genital orifice, thus birth can be termed a 'breech case'. Females always select shaded sites for larviposition. The larva is deposited on loose friable soil, sand or humus, frequently underneath bushes, trees, fallen logs, rocks, between buttress roots of trees, in sandy river beds, in animal burrows and even in rot holes in trees which may be formed some distance above the ground (4–5 m). Immediately the larva is deposited it commences to bury under 2–5 cm of soil. After about 15 minutes the 3rd-instar larval

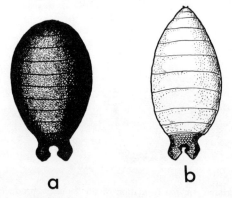

a   b

Fig. 8.5 Tsetse fly. (a) puparium; (b) larva.

skin contracts and hardens to form a reddish-brown or dark brown, barrel-shaped puparium which is about 5–8 mm long and has distinct polypneustic lobes (Fig. 8.5a). Within this puparial case the larva pupates.

The duration of the pupal period is comparatively long, usually extending over 4–5 weeks but at high temperatures may be completed within 3 weeks, and conversely at low temperatures prolonged to 13 weeks. After pupal development has been completed the fly emerges from the puparium, forces its way to the surface of the ground and flies away.

During the development of the larva within the female the tsetse feeds several times, about once every 2–3 days. The first larva is deposited about 16–20 days after the female has emerged from the puparium, thereafter, if food is plentiful a larva is deposited about every 9–12 days. In the laboratory female tsetse flies have produced up to 20 offspring but the average is nearer 5–8. Breeding generally continues throughout the year but in very humid conditions reproduction may be diminished. Maximum population size is usually obtained at the end of the rainy season. The population diminishes in the dry season when suitable areas of refuge for adult flies and suitable larviposition sites may become restricted and localised.

Adult behaviour

Knowledge of certain aspects of the behaviour of tsetse flies is essential for an understanding of approaches to their control, and also the part vector species play in the transmission of sleeping sickness.

Blood-engorged tsetse flies, and unfed hungry flies waiting to feed on suitable hosts, spend the nights and much of the daytime hours resting in dark and usually humid resting sites. During the day the favoured resting sites of most species are twigs, branches and trunks of trees and bushes. Flies are not found resting in sites in which temperatures rise above about 36 °C. At night tsetse flies prefer to rest on the upper surfaces of leaves. Accurate knowledge of the actual resting sites may be required for control measures. For example, the height at which adults rest on trees determines the height at which the trees need to be sprayed with insecticides. Most species in fact rest below 4 m; in Nigeria 50 per cent of

G. palpalis and *G. morsitans* commonly rest between ground level and 30 cm.

Based on their morphology, ecology, karyotype and behaviour tsetses can be separated into the following three main groups.

Fusca *group (forest flies)*

This group contains 14 species and subspecies of *Glossina*, all of which are large (10·5–15·5 mm). They are forest flies (except *G. longipennis*) and most are restricted to the equatorial forests of West and Central Africa, for example *G. fusca* occurs in relict forests of West and Central Africa and *G. brevipalpis* in secondary forests of East Africa.

The *fusca* group rarely feeds on man and none of the species is a vector of sleeping sickness.

Morsitans *group (savanna flies)*

Seven species and subspecies are included within this group. They are medium sized insects, 7·5–11 mm long and typically inhabit the savanna regions of Africa, which may extend from the coast, or the edges of forests to dry semi-desert regions. *Glossina morsitans* occupies the savanna regions of West, Central and East Africa, whereas *G. pallidipes* and *G. swynnertoni* are restricted to the savannas of East Africa. The former two species occur in country ranging from wooded savanna at the edges of forests to the dry thicket vegetation of arid regions, while *G. swynnertoni* is mainly restricted to relatively dry thicket country.

All three species above are vectors of sleeping sickness, the most important being *G. morsitans*.

Palpalis *group (riverine and forest flies)*

Nine tsetse species and subspecies are found in this group, the smallest being about 6·5 mm in length and the largest 11 mm. They are essentially flies inhabiting wetter types of vegetation, such as forests, luxuriant scrub and vegetation growing along rivers and shores of lakes. *Glossina palpalis* inhabits riverine vegetation bordering rivers and lakes, mangrove swamps and forested areas, and occurs throughout most of West Africa, down

the western part of the continent to Angola. *Glossina fuscipes,*
which is closely related to *G. palpalis,* occurs mainly in Central
Africa but extends its range to the western areas of East Africa.
Glossina tachinoides is a riverine species found near streams and
rivers in wet humid coastal areas, through wooded savanna regions to the riverine vegetation of very dry savanna areas. It is
found mainly in West and Central Africa but also occurs in
Ethiopia.

All these species are vectors of sleeping sickness.

MEDICAL IMPORTANCE

Probably any species of tsetse fly can transmit African trypanosomiasis to man. In practice, however, relatively few species of
tsetse flies are natural vectors because many species rarely, if ever,
feed on man. It is the behaviour of the adult tsetse and the degree
of fly–man contact, and in the case of Rhodesian sleeping sickness
it is also the degree of vector contact with the reservoir hosts of
the trypanosomes, that establishes whether a tsetse fly is a vector.

Sleeping sickness has a patchy distribution over about 10^6 km^2
of land in Africa; about 10 000 new cases are detected annually.
There are two subspecies (sometimes regarded as distinct species)
of trypanosomes causing African sleeping sickness in man, *Trypanosoma brucei gambiense* and *T. brucei rhodesiense.* These parasites are morphologically indistinguishable but produce different clinical symptoms in man and have different epidemiologies.
The most important vectors of sleeping sickness are *G. palpalis,*
G. fuscipes, *G. tachinoides,* *G. morsitans,* *G. pallidipes* and *G.
swynnertoni.*

The cycle of development of *Trypanosoma brucei gambiense* and
T. brucei rhodesiense in the tsetse fly is the same and is as follows.
Trypanosomes (amastigotes) sucked up by male or female tsetse
flies during a blood-meal from an infected man (or in the case of
T. brucei rhodesiense mainly from a non-human reservoir) pass
first through the oesophagus to the crop, and then after feeding
has ceased, into the peritrophic tube lining the mid gut. Blood
is digested within the mid gut. However, the *gambiense* and
rhodesiense trypanosomes are not destroyed but in fact multiply.
There is still some uncertainty as to the exact migratory route

the trypanosomes take to reach the fly's salivary glands. Until recently it was believed that the only way in which they could infect the salivary glands was for them to travel round the end of the peritrophic membrane and migrate between it and the mid gut wall back to the proventriculus. Here the peritrophic membrane is soft and more or less fluid which allows the parasites to penetrate it and pass to the oesophagus, from here they continue their journey through the pharynx down to the tip of the proboscis. They then migrate up the salivary duct in the hypopharynx to reach the paired salivary glands where the mature infective metacyclic forms (trypomastigotes) develop. These are injected into the host when the fly feeds. The interval between the time a tsetse fly engorges on an infected person to that when its salivary glands contain infective trypanosomes varies between 18–34 days. More recently, however, it has been found that *T. brucei rhodesiense* parasites in *Glossina morsitans* can penetrate the gut cells and pass across into the haemocele, from where it seems they can migrate directly to the salivary glands. The importance of this more direct route of trypanosomal migration to the salivary glands is as yet unclear.

When establishing infection rates in tsetse flies by dissection, any trypanosomes found in the gut or proboscis are ignored as only those in the salivary glands can be ascribed with any degree of certaintly to *T. brucei gambiense* or *T. brucei rhodesiense*, but there are complications: *T. brucei brucei*, which does not cause sleeping sickness in man but causes an animal trypanosomiasis commonly called nagana, undergoes a similar cyclical development in the fly. Consequently, the presence of trypomastigotes (metacyclic forms) in the salivary glands does not necessarily indicate infection of trypanosomes infective to man.

Salivary gland infection rates in tsetse flies are low, nearly always being less than 1 per cent, even in areas of endemic sleeping sickness.

Gambian sleeping sickness

Glossina palpalis and *G. tachinoides* are the most important vectors in West Africa, and *G. fuscipes* is, in Central and East Africa, of *T. brucei gambiense*, the causative agent of Gambian sleeping sickness. This disease is relatively chronic, with death often not occurring until after many years. Until recently it was considered that there were no natural reservoirs of the disease other than man, but studies in West Africa indicate that domestic pigs and some wild mammals may harbour *T. brucei gambiense*.

The vectors of Gambian sleeping sickness are especially common at watering places, fords across rivers and along lake shores etc., in fact in places where people frequently visit to collect water or do their washing. As a consequence there may be limited and localised foci of transmission.

Rhodesian sleeping sickness

The causative agent, *T. brucei rhodesiense*, causes a more virulent disease than *T. brucei gambiense* but it is not so widespread, being more or less restricted to Tanzania, Malawi, Zambia, Zimbabwe, Mozambique and to the northern areas of Lake Victoria in Kenya and Uganda. The most important vectors are *G. morsitans*, *G. swynnertoni* and *G. pallidipes*, species which feed on a variety of game animals and domestic livestock, especially bovids, in preference to man. These flies often occur in savanna areas thinly populated by humans. Wild animals, especially a number of bovid species, are important reservoirs of *T. brucei rhodesiense*. The disease is a zoonosis.

CONTROL

Because the immature stages are so well protected, the larva being retained by the female for almost all of its life, and the puparium being buried in the soil, control against tsetse flies is aimed at the adults.

Many control methods have been directed at tsetse flies to combat human and animal trypanosomiasis. At one time there were campaigns in Zimbabwe and some East African countries to kill in selected areas all game animals that might provide food for tsetses, or be reservoirs of trypanosomiasis. The wide scale and often indiscriminate slaughter of animals is no longer acceptable in a world that is increasingly sensitive to the preservation of wild-life.

The distribution and abundance of tsetse flies is largely determined by types of vegetation and microclimate; their dependence on such requirements gave rise to another form of control. This consisted of clearing vegetation, especially that near rivers and lake shores, either completely or partially, and often on a large scale so that habitats were opened up and made unsuitable for tsetses. The destruction of such vegetation has in the past achieved considerable success in controlling tsetse flies, but in many countries this method, at least on a large scale, is at present no longer ecologically or economically acceptable. However, it may in the future again play a part in control, especially in an integrated approach.

There are no problems of insecticide resistance with tsetse flies, and at present tsetse control relies almost exclusively on insecticides. Persistent organochlorine insecticides such as DDT and dieldrin can be applied as either wettable powders or emulsions to vegetation harbouring adults. The success of such methods depends on a detailed knowledge of the behaviour and resting sites of the vectors. For example, it is often possible to restrict spraying to tree trunks up to a height of 1·5 m during the dry season, extending this to 3·5 m in the wet season. Insecticides are often sprayed on vegetation at concentrations of 1·5–5 per cent active ingredient, either from knapsack sprayers or from other ground-based machines. The frequency of application depends much on local conditions, such as rainfall, other climatic factors and the growth and spread of fresh vegetation which can provide new resting sites free of insecticides.

Alternatively, aerial applications of insecticides can be made. For example, ultra-low-volume dosages of non-residual formulations of endosulfan or synthetic pyrethroids like deltamethrin, from fixed-wing aircraft, or as residual deposits of dieldrin and endosulfan applied from helicopters. Although aerial spraying, particularly of residual deposits, results in a greater coverage of vegetation by the insecticides than achieved by ground application techniques, it usually kills a greater number of non-target insects and animals, many of which may be directly or indirectly beneficial to man. Repeated applications, especially of non-residual insecticides like the synthetic pyrethroids, are necessary because the tsetse population is in the soil as puparia for 4–5 weeks or longer, and so is not affected by spraying. There is no doubt that indiscriminate or intensive and repeated spraying of residual organochlorine insecticides can have disastrous effects on the local fauna, but it should be appreciated that the application rates of insecticides for tsetse control are often very low. It should also be realised that after tsetse flies have been eradicated from an area and spraying stopped, many, if not all, of the wild-life populations may revert to their original size. Intensive bush clearance for tsetse control can also greatly diminish the numbers and variety of local fauna, but in this instance the change may be permanent, especially if local people occupy and farm areas that were originally scrub or forest.

Chapter 9
Houseflies and Stableflies

There are many genera and species of flies belonging to the family Muscidae. The most important from the medical aspect are the common housefly, other houseflies, the latrine fly and the blood-sucking stablefly. All these flies have a more or less world-wide distribution. The non-biting flies, such as the houseflies and the latrine flies, are vectors of cestodes, nematodes, faecal bacteria, protozoa and viruses, resulting in the spread of such enteric diseases as the dysenteries and typhoids. The stablefly can be a mechanical vector of trypanosomiasis.

THE COMMON HOUSEFLY *MUSCA DOMESTICA*

External morphology

Houseflies have a world-wide distribution. They are medium sized non-metallic flies about 6–9 mm in length, varying in colour from light to dark grey. They have four broadish dorsal, dark longitudinal stripes on the thorax (Fig. 9.1a). The antennae consist of three segments, the last and biggest of which is cylindrical and has a prominent hair, called an arista, which has hairs on both sides. The antennae are concealed in depressions on the front of the face of the fly and are not easily seen. The mouthparts (proboscis) of the housefly are complicated and specially adapted for sucking up fluid or semi-fluid foods. When not in use they are partially withdrawn into the head capsule (Fig. 9.2a), but are extended vertically downwards in a telescopic fashion when the fly feeds. The proboscis ends in a pair of oval-shaped fleshy labellae, having very fine channels called pseudotracheae through which fluids can be sucked up. Houseflies feed on a great variety of substances, such as sugar, milk, almost all food of man, rotting vegetables and carcasses, excreta and vomit, in fact almost any organic material. The method of feeding differs according to the

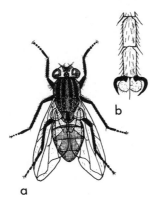

Fig. 9.1 *Musca domestica.* (a) Adult fly; (b) terminal tarsal segments showing paired claws, paired pulvilli and single bristle-like empodium.

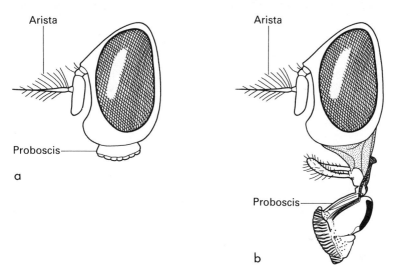

Fig. 9.2 Lateral views of head of *M. domestica.* (a) Proboscis retracted; (b) proboscis extended for feeding.

physical state of the food. For example, for thin fluids, such as milk and beer, the labellae are closely appressed on to the food which is then sucked up through the small openings in the pseudotracheae. When feeding on semi-solids like excreta, sputum, and nasal discharges, the labellae are completely everted and food is sucked up directly into a food channel formed by the apposition of the slender labrum and blade-like hypopharynx. If flies feed on more solid materials such as sugar lumps, dried blood, cheese and cooked meats, the labellae are everted and minute prestomal teeth surrounding the food channel are exposed and scrape away at the solid food. The fly then moistens small particles with either saliva or the regurgitated contents of its crop, after which the food is sucked up. This latter type of feeding is clearly a method which is conducive to the spread of a variety of pathogens.

The wings of the housefly have vein 4 bending up sharply to join the costa close to vein 3 (Fig. 9.3). This is an important taxonomic character which can help distinguish *Musca* species from other rather similar flies. Each of three pairs of legs end in a pair of claws and a pair of fleshy pad-like structures called the pulvilli, which are supplied with glandular hairs (see Fig. 9.1b). These sticky hairs enable the fly to adhere to very smooth surfaces, such as windows, and are also responsible for the fly picking

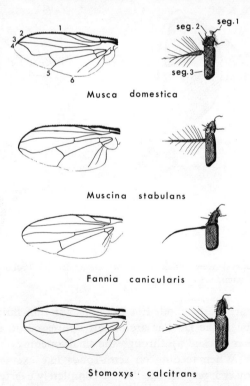

Fig. 9.3 Wing venation and antenna characteristic of the genera *Musca*, *Muscina*, *Fannia* and *Stomoxys*. Note endings of veins 3 and 4.

up dirt and pathogens when it visits excreta, septic wounds, rubbish dumps, etc. There are four visible greyish abdominal segments which are usually partially obscured from view by the wings.

Life-cycle

Female *Musca domestica* are attracted to a variety of decomposing materials for egg laying, such as horse manure, poultry dung, urine-contaminated bedding, foodstuff, carcasses, decomposing organic materials found in rubbish dumps, household garbage and waste foods from kitchens and hotels. During egg laying 75–100 eggs are deposited together, or in separate batches, either in cracks and crevices or scattered over the surface. A fly may deposit five or six such egg batches in her lifetime. The eggs are creamy-white, about 0·8–1·2 mm long, and distinctly concave dorsally giving them a banana-shaped appearance (Fig. 9.4a). They can hatch after only 6–12 hours, but this period is extended in cool weather. Hatching is accomplished by the strip of egg shell between parallel ridges on the dorsal concave surface lifting up, and partially detaching itself from the rest of the egg. Eggs cannot withstand desiccation and die if they dry out. Neither can they tolerate extremes of temperatures, most dying after exposure to temperatures below 15°C or above 40°C.

The creamy-white larvae which hatch from the eggs are 12-segmented, cylindrical and maggot-shaped (Fig. 9.4b). There are no spicules covering the body. At the pointed head end there is

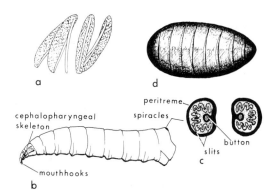

Fig. 9.4 *Musca domestica*. (a) Eggs; (b) larva; (c) posterior D-shaped larval spiracles; (d) puparium.

a pair of small curved mouthhooks, which are seen as a blackish structure situated beneath the integument of the head and first few thoracic segments. At the posterior end of the body there is a pair of conspicuous spiracles shaped like a letter D. Each spiracle has a complete and thick outer wall called the peritreme which encloses three very sinuous spiracular slits (Fig. 9.4c).

Larvae feed on liquid food resulting from decomposing and decaying organic material. There are three larval instars. Mature larvae measure about 8–14 mm, the final size depending on environmental conditions, especially the amount of available food. The speed of larval growth and development depends on the abundance of food supply and temperature. Development may be completed within only 3–5 days, but under less favourable conditions 7–10 days are needed, and in cool weather development may extend to about 24 days.

If larval habitats dry out the larvae are killed, but if they become too wet they drown.

Prior to pupation the 3rd-instar larvae may migrate away from their larval habitats to drier ground. Sometimes, however, the periphery of breeding places, such as rubbish dumps, may be sufficiently dry for larvae to pupate there; pupation may also occur in the dry soil underneath larval habitats. Pupation begins with the larval skin contracting, hardening and turning dark brown, after which a barrel-shaped structure measuring about 6 mm, called a puparium, is formed. Close examination shows this is segmented (Fig. 9.4d). The puparium is often referred to as the pupa but technically this is incorrect because the actual pupa is formed within the protective shell of the puparial case. (A puparium is also formed by tsetse flies; see Chapter 8.) The puparial stage lasts about 3–5 days in warm weather, but may be prolonged to 7–14 days during cooler periods.

Developmental time from egg to adult is about 49 days at 16°C, 21 days at 20°C, 16 days at 23°C, 9–11 days at 30°C and 8 days at 35°C. Occasionally the period can be less than 7 days. In temperate areas a varying, but usually small, proportion of houseflies may survive throughout the winter as puparia, but more frequently they overwinter as hibernating adults. Occasionally there is very prolonged but continuous larval development during the winter months.

The adult fly escapes from its puparial case by pushing off its anterior end, crawling out and flying away.

Adults of *Musca domestica* generally avoid direct sunlight, preferring to seek shelter in buildings inhabited by man or his animals. Houseflies and related flies, and the calliphorid flies discussed in the next chapter, are often called domestic or synanthropic flies, because of their close association with man and his home. Houseflies defecate at random, and frequently regurgitate their foods, resulting in unsightly 'fly spots'. Adults frequently fly 3–4 km from their emergence sites, and may travel as far as 34 km.

Other species of houseflies

There are about 60 species and subspecies of *Musca*, all of which, except *M. domestica* which is widespread in its distribution, and *M. autumnalis*, which occurs both in the Old and New Worlds, are confined to the Old World.

Musca sorbens is abundant in the tropics and subtropics of the Old World. It is very similar to *Musca domestica* but is more rarely found indoors and prefers light to shaded places, and has a greater tolerance to high temperatures. Adults are more attracted to the human body than *M. domestica*. They are especially common on the face, around the eyes, on sores and on any discharges. Females mature up to about 80 eggs at a time and these are laid in one or several batches, especially on human excrement, but excreta of other animals such as pigs, cows and dogs, and also carcasses, provide suitable larval habitats. At 25–28°C the life-cycle from egg to adult takes about 9 days.

Medical importance

Houseflies can transmit a large number of diseases to man owing to their habits of visiting, almost indiscriminately, faeces and other unhygienic matter and man's food. Pathogens are spread by the flies' contaminated feet, body hairs and mouthparts. In addition, they vomit during feeding and frequently defecate on food. Over 100 different pathogens have been recorded from houseflies, at least 65 of which are known to be transmitted. Transmission is mechanical, that is, the fly acts as a physical carrier. None of the pathogens undergoes obligatory cyclical development in the fly.

Houseflies can transmit viruses such as poliomyelitis, trachoma,

Coxsackie virus and infectious hepatitis, as well as rickettsiae such as Q fever (*Coxiella burneti*), and numerous bacterial diseases, but mainly enteric ones such as bacillary dysentery (*Shigella*), cholera, the typhoids and paratyphoids (*Salmonella*). A variety of streptococci and staphylococci, conjunctivitis, yaws, and more rarely even tuberculosis, leprosy and anthrax can be spread by flies. They may also be vectors of protozoan parasites such as the amoebic dysenteries (*Entamoeba, Giardia*). In addition, they may carry eggs of a variety of tapeworms, for example, *Taenia* spp. including *T. solium, Hymenolepis nana, H. diminuta, Dipylidium caninum, Diphyllobothrium latum* and several others, also nematodes such as *Necator, Ancylostoma, Thelazia californiensis, Tricocephalus trichiurus, Enterobius vermicularis* and *Ascaris lumbricoides*. Furthermore, they can be carriers in the tropical Americas of the eggs of *Dermatobia hominis*, a myiasis-producing fly (see Chapter 10).

Larvae of houseflies have occasionally been recorded in cases of urinogenital and traumatic myiasis, and more rarely in aural and nasopharyngeal myiasis. If food infected with fly maggots is eaten, then they may be passed more or less intact in the excreta, often causing considerable alarm and surprise. There is, however, no true intestinal myiasis in man (see Chapter 10).

Because of their dirty habits houseflies are potential vectors of many pathogens to man, but it is difficult to assess their relative importance in the transmission of most diseases. Much information of their real role in the spread of disease is circumstantial, for example, seasonal increase of fly abundance is often closely correlated with outbreaks of diarrhoeal diseases. The classic demonstration of the association between flies and disease was in two Texas towns in 1946 and 1947. One town was sprayed with DDT to destroy the houseflies; this was accompanied by a reduced incidence of *Shigella* infections and a marked decrease in the number of deaths in children due to diarrhoea. The unsprayed town did not have such a reduction in *Shigella* infections. A similar association between the incidence of diarrhoea and housefly abundance has been observed in Palestinian refugee camps.

Control

Control methods can be divided conveniently into three categories.

1 Physical and mechanical
2 Environmental sanitation
3 Insecticidal

Physical and mechanical control

Flies and other obnoxious insects can sometimes be prevented from entering buildings by screening windows, openings, air vents, etc. Screens should be made of non-corrosive material, such as plastic, copper or aluminium gauze, and have a mesh size of 3–4 strands per centimetre. This will exclude relatively large insects such as houseflies from buildings, without unduly decreasing air circulation or light. Screening can be costly, but may be worthwhile employing in hospitals and restaurants. It may be unnecessary to screen windows higher than the fourth floor of buildings. Screening should be periodically inspected and any tears mended. Screening can reduce fly nuisance but does not solve the problem, for flies will continue to breed locally and to enter unscreened houses.

The establishment in doorways of an air current, such as the air barriers found in the entrances of some shops, and fans mounted over doorways may help to reduce the number of flies entering premises. The well-known practice of placing in doorways curtains made of many vertical, often coloured, strips of plastic or beading also helps to keep out flies. A not uncommon method, especially in restaurants and food stores, is to mount an ultraviolet light trap on a wall. Flies attracted to the trap are electrocuted on entering it by contact with an electric grid.

Environmental sanitation

Environmental sanitation aims at drastically curtailing housefly populations by reducing their breeding places. For example, domestic refuse and garbage should be placed in either strong plastic bags and the openings tightly closed, or in dustbins with tight-fitting lids. When possible there should also be regular refuse collections, preferably twice a week in warm countries, to prevent any eggs laid amongst the garbage developing into adults. If household refuse cannot be collected it should be burnt or buried. Unhygienic rubbish dumps, so commonly found in towns and villages, provide ideal breeding places for houseflies, and should be abolished. Refuse should be placed in pits which are covered, daily if possible, with a 15-cm layer of earth; when the pits are more or less full they must be finally covered with 60 cm of compacted earth. This depth of final fill is required to prevent rodents being attracted to buried decomposing organic material and burrowing into the rubbish pits.

It is also important to organise efficient disposal of household and industrial sewage and sanitary wastes. There should also be efficient latrines which prevent the breeding of houseflies and allied flies.

Insecticidal control

Many different types of insecticides and procedures have been used to reduce fly nuisances. Commercially available small aerosol dispensers are commonly used in homes as space-sprays to kill flies. Most of these aerosols contain knock-down insecticides such as 0·5 per cent dichlorvos (DDVP) or 0·1–0·2 per cent pyrethrins synergised with piperonyl butoxide. Synthetic pyrethroids used as a 0·1 per cent spray need no synergists and are 20 times more toxic to houseflies than natural pyrethrins. Aerosol sprays have virtually no residual effect and consequently must be repeatedly used to achieve control; they do little to alleviate the source of the fly nuisance, and moreover they can be costly.

The outdoor application of insecticidal aerosols or mists from special spraying machines can give effective control in certain situations, such as in and around dairies, farms and poultry sheds. Organophosphate insecticides such as malathion, diazinon, fenthion (Baytex), naled (Dibrom) and dichlorvos (DDVP) have been successfully used in outdoor aerosol applications.

Flies may also be controlled by spraying the indoor walls, ceilings, doors, etc. with residual insecticides such as 3 per cent malathion, 1 per cent dimethoate, 0·5–1·0 per cent fenchlorphos (Ronnel), 1–2 per cent tetrachlorvinphos (Rabon) or 1 per cent propoxur (Baygon). These residual insecticides should remain effective for 1–2 months, but much depends on local circumstances and whether walls are washed. The outside walls of houses and cattle sheds may also be sprayed with residual insecticides, but their duration of effectiveness will depend on several factors, such as whether the surface deposit is washed off by rain, or rubbed off.

Alternative methods employ strips of cord or rope soaked in such insecticides as diazinon and dyed, preferably red, to alert people that it is impregnated with insecticides. Flies are killed when they rest on these cords hung up in dairies and houses. Dichlorvos resin strips are also commonly used to control flies in houses, restaurants, hotel kitchens, dairies, etc. These impregnated strips kill flies by dissemination of the dichlorvos vapour. They may remain effective for 2–3 months, but this depends on the temperature and degree of ventilation in the rooms in which they are used.

Insecticides can also be directed against the larvae, such as spraying the insides and outsides of dustbins and the walls adjacent to them with emulsions of 0·5 per cent diazinon or 0·5 per cent malathion. Refuse and garbage heaps, manure piles and other large breeding sites can be sprayed with a variety of insecticides, but the main problem is that there is usually insufficient penetration of insecticide into these breeding places to give effective control. However, regular spraying of such piles of breeding media may deter flies from settling on them and ovipositing, and may even kill some adult flies.

Attractant fly baits have also been used to control houseflies. Sugar mixed with an inert carrier such as sand or bran and treated with 1–2 per cent insecticides provides an attractive solid bait. Liquid baits commonly comprise 10 per cent sugar dissolved in water plus 0·1–0·2 per cent insecticides. The most commonly used insecticides in both dry and liquid baits are malathion, diazinon, dichlorvos, naled (Dibrom) or fenchlorphos (Ronnel), either alone or in combination. In some countries commercially prepared dry or liquid baits are available. Dry baits can be scattered or placed in wooden, plastic or metal trays. Liquid baits can be placed in a glass bottle which is inverted over a saucer-like receptacle so that as the bait evaporates in the receptacle more flows in from the reservoir, as in automatic water feeders for poultry. Attractant baits can very quickly produce spectacular reductions of flies in buildings, but solid baits must be replaced about every 2 days.

In many parts of the world houseflies have become resistant to many of the more commonly used organochlorine and organophosphate insecticides, and also unfortunately to the synthetic pyrethroids.

FANNIA SPECIES

External morphology

Flies of the genus *Fannia* resemble houseflies but are rather smaller (6–7 mm), and are readily distinguished from houseflies and other similar flies by their wing venation and antennae (see Fig. 9.3). In *Fannia* vein 4 of the wing is more or less parallel to vein 3, whereas in *Musca* it bends upwards and almost touches vein 3 at the wing apex, while in *Muscina* vein 4 also bends upwards but not to such an extent. The arista, which arises from the third antennal segment, is completely devoid of hairs (see Fig. 9.3), whereas in both *Musca* and *Muscina* it bears branches on both sides. In most other respects the adult flies are similar to houseflies. There are two common species of *Fannia* which are of minor medical importance, namely *Fannia canicularis* (the lesser housefly) which occurs world-wide and is commonly encountered in houses, and *Fannia scalaris* (the latrine fly) which has a Holarctic distribution and is less common in houses. *F. canicularis* has three longitudinal stripes on the thorax, while *F. scalaris* has two such stripes.

Life-cycle

The lesser housefly (*M. canicularis*) lays about 50–100 eggs, which resemble those of the common housefly. They are deposited on man's food, but but also on urine-soaked bedding of man and animals, compost heaps, decaying piles of grass, human and animal excreta and in poultry litter. The latrine fly (*M. scalaris*) usually lays her eggs on faeces—hence the name.

Eggs hatch after 1–2 days. *Fannia* larvae are quite distinct from the maggot-shaped larvae of *Musca* and are unlikely to be confused with the larvae of any other medically important fly (Fig. 9.5). They are flattened dorsoventrally and have many thin but conspicuous fleshy processes arising from the body segments which bear small spiniform secondary processes. Larval development takes about 7–12 days but may be prolonged if the habitat

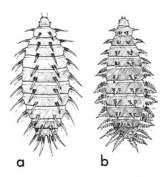

Fig. 9.5 Larvae. (a) *Fannia canicularis*; (b) *Fannia scalaris*.

starts to dry out. The puparium is brown in colour and is similar
to the shape of the larva. After 7–10 days the adult fly emerges.
The life-cycle often lasts about 1 month which is considerably
longer than in *Musca domestica*, but may under favourable conditions be completed within 13–22 days. The feeding mechanism
of the adult is similar to that of *M. domestica*. Although *Fannia*
adults often enter houses they do not settle on man, or on his
food, as much as houseflies.

Medical importance

Many of the pathogens transmitted by the housefly are probably
also spread by *Fannia* species. They have been incriminated in
cases of urinogenital myiasis, and larvae are sometimes found in
stools, but as previously stressed true intestinal myiasis does not
occur in man.

Control

The same methods apply to species of *Fannia* as to *Musca*, but
particular attention should be given to the prevention and eradication of *Fannia scalaris* breeding in latrines.

THE GREATER HOUSEFLY (*MUSCINA STABULANS*)

External morphology

Muscina stabulans has a world-wide distribution and is commonly referred to as the greater housefly. Adults are about 7–10 mm long, slightly larger than houseflies. They can be distinguished from both *Musca* and *Fannia* because vein 4 of the wing curves slightly, but distinctly, upwards towards vein 3 (Fig. 9.3), and from *Fannia*, but not *Musca*, by having hairs on both the upper and lower sides of the arista (see Fig. 9.3).

Life-cycle

Females scatter about 150–200 eggs more or less indiscriminately over the surface of decaying matter such as rotting fruits, vegetables and fungi, on cooked and raw meats especially if putrified, on carcasses and also on human and animal excreta. The eggs hatch after 1–2 days and the resultant larvae resemble the maggot-shaped larvae of the housefly, but can be distinguished by the structure of the posterior spiracles. In *M. stabulans* the spiracles are almost circular, not D-shaped as in *M. domestica*. Furthermore, the peritreme, which is very wide, encircles three crescent-shaped spiracular slits (Fig. 9.6b). Young larvae are omnivorous scavengers, as are larvae of *Musca* and *Fannia*, but towards the end of the larval period they become predacious, feeding on any other fly larvae in the breeding places. The brown puparium is similar in shape to that of *M. domestica* and its duration is about 1–2 weeks. Like *Fannia* species the life-cycle is about 4–6 weeks, although in warm weather it may be reduced to 20–25 days.

Adults enter buildings and feed and behave much the same as do adults of *M. domestica*.

Medical importance

The exact role of *M. stabulans* as a disease vector remains undetermined, but many of the pathogens transmitted by the housefly are probably also spread by *Muscina*. Larvae, like those of *Fannia* and *Musca*, have occasionally been recorded in cases of accidental intestinal myiasis.

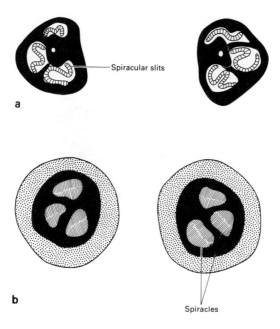

Fig. 9.6   Posterior larval spiracles. (a) *Stomoxys calcitrans*; (b) *Muscina stabulans*.

Control

The control measures are very similar to those applied to the housefly.

THE STABLEFLY (*STOMOXYS CALCITRANS*)

External morphology

Stableflies have a world-wide distribution. They are sometimes known as the biting housefly or dogfly. The most common species is *Stomoxys calcitrans*. Adults have four black longitudinal stripes on a dark grey thorax and are about the same size (5–6 mm) as houseflies, which they superficially resemble. They are, however,

easily separated from *Musca*, *Fannia* and *Muscina* by a conspicuous forward projecting, rigid proboscis (Fig. 9.7). The wing
venation resembles that of *Muscina*. The arista of the third antennal segment differs from *Musca*, *Fannia* and *Muscina* in having
hairs arising from only the upper side (see Fig. 9.3).

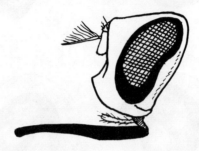

Fig. 9.7 Lateral view of head of *Stomoxys calcitrans* showing forwardly directed
proboscis.

In Africa adults might at first glance be confused with tsetse
flies which also have a forward projecting proboscis, but *Stomoxys
calcitrans* is a smaller fly. Also, when at rest its wings are not
placed completely over the body in a closed scissor-like fashion
as in tsetse flies, but are kept apart as in houseflies. Furthermore,
there is no enclosed hatchet cell in the wings, as found in tsetse
flies.

Life-cycle

Both males and females take blood-meals from wild and domesticated animals, including cattle, horses, pigs and dogs; they also
feed on man, especially if their more preferred hosts are absent
or scarce in the area. Their bites can be painful and most are on
the legs. During feeding the forward projecting proboscis is
swung downwards, and the skin penetrated. In hot weather, flies
digest their blood-meals within 12–24 hours and feed about every
1–3 days, but in cooler conditions blood digestion is prolonged to
2–4 days or more, and feeding occurs every 5–10 days. Biting is
restricted to the daylight hours and occurs both in bright sunshine and cloudy overcast weather. Most biting occurs outdoors

but stableflies will also enter houses to feed. They are mostly encountered in and around farms or where horses are kept, and consequently are more common in rural areas than in towns.

The creamy-white eggs, 1 mm long, resemble those of houseflies. They are normally laid in batches of less than 20, but sometimes as many as 50–100 may be laid together. Eggs are usually deposited in horse manure but also in compost pits, decaying and fermenting piles of vegetable matter, weeds, cut grass or hay. Stableflies very rarely lay their eggs in human or animal faeces, unless it is liberally mixed with hay or straw.

Eggs hatch within 1–4 days. The resultant larvae are creamy-coloured maggots which resemble those of the housefly. However, they can be separated by the arrangement of the posterior spiracles, which are widely separated (see Fig. 9.6a), thus differing from the more closely positioned spiracular plates of *Musca* and *Muscina*. They are also approximately round in outline, lack a peritreme, and the S-shaped spiracles are widely separated from each other. Larvae prefer a high degree of moisture for development and therefore are found mostly in wet mixtures of manure and soil or straw, and in vegetable matter in advanced stages of decay. Under optimum conditions the larval period lasts about 6–10 days, but in cooler weather, or when there is a shortage of food, larval development can be prolonged to 4–5 weeks or more.

Larvae migrate to drier areas and bury themselves in the soil prior to pupation. The puparium is dark brown and resembles that of the housefly, but can be distinguished from it by having the posterior spiracles widely separated. The puparial stage lasts 5–26 days. The life-cycle from egg laying to adult emergence may last from 12 to 58 days, the time depending mainly on temperature.

In tropical areas stableflies breed continuously throughout the year, but in more temperate climates they pass through the cooler months as larvae or puparia. Sometimes adults survive winters in warm stables or buildings, feeding intermittently during the cooler months.

Medical importance

Because of the painful bites inflicted by both sexes stableflies can be serious pests of man and cattle. Adult flies are not regarded as transmitting diseases to man, although under certain conditions they can be mechanical vectors of human (and animal) trypano-somiasis, but their role in spreading trypanosomiasis is minimal, except for *T. evansi*, the causative agent of Surra, which infects camels, horses and other mammals. Because stableflies rarely visit excreta and festering wounds they are much less likely to spread pathogens in the way houseflies do.

In the tropical Americas eggs of *Dermatobia hominis*, a myiasis-producing fly (see Chapter 10), are sometimes attached to adult stableflies.

Control

Many of the control methods aimed at houseflies can be applied with some modification to control stableflies. For example, not allowing piles of manure, grass cuttings or decaying vegetable matter to accumulate, and burning straw and bedding material. Breeding places can be sprayed with organochlorine or organo-phosphate insecticides, but as noted in the section on housefly control it is difficult to get deep insecticidal penetration into the breeding places where most larvae are found. Insecticidal spray-ing of horse stables, animal shelters, barns and other farm build-ings can help reduce their numbers.

Chapter 10
Flies and Myiasis

Myiasis can be defined as the invasion of organs and tissues of man or other vertebrate animals with *dipterous* larvae, which for at least a period feed upon the living, necrotic or dead tissues, or in the case of intestinal myiasis, on the host's ingested food. Different terms can be used to describe myiasis which affects different parts of the body, for example: cutaneous, dermal or subdermal myiasis; urinogenital myiasis; ophthalmic myiasis; nasopharyngeal myiasis; and intestinal or enteric myiasis. When larvae burrow just under the surface layers of the skin this is sometimes called creeping eruption or creeping myiasis; when boil-like lesions are produced the term furuncular myiasis may be used, and when wounds become infested this is often referred to as traumatic myiasis.

Myiasis may be obligatory or facultative. In obligatory myiasis it is essential for the fly larvae to live on a live host for at least a certain part of their life. For example, larvae of *Cordylobia anthropophaga*, *Cochliomyia hominivorax*, *Chrysomya bezziana*, *Dermatobia hominis*, and *Wohlfahrtia* are obligatory parasites of man and other vertebrates. In contrast, in facultative myiasis larvae are normally free-living, often attacking carcasses, but under certain conditions they may infect living hosts. Several types of fly, including species of *Calliphora*, *Lucilia*, *Phormia* and *Sarcophaga*, which normally breed in meat or carrion, may cause facultative cutaneous myiasis in man by infecting festering sores and wounds.

There is no obligatory intestinal myiasis of man. When man has maggots in his intestinal tract this is most likely due to accidental swallowing of eggs or larvae on food. Although the maggots may be able to survive for some time in the intestine, there is no species of fly which is specially adapted to cause intestinal myiasis in man. In contrast, obligatory intestinal myiasis occurs in animals. The presence of larvae in man's intestine may nevertheless cause considerable discomfort, abdominal pain and

155

diarrhoea, which may be accompanied by discharge of blood and vomiting. Living larvae may be passed with the excreta or vomit. Occasionally facultative urinogenital myiasis occurs in man—this usually involves larvae of *Musca* or *Fannia* species. It seems that ovipositing flies are attracted to unhygienic discharges and lay their eggs near genital orifices. When these eggs hatch the minute larvae enter the genital orifice and work their way up the urogenital tract. Much pain may be caused by larvae obstructing these passages, and mucous and blood, and eventually larvae, may be discharged with the urine.

When larvae occur in wounds, sores and dermal or subdermal tissues, their removal under asceptic conditions is usually a relatively simple procedure. When they are more deeply imbedded in the underlying tissues, or when they have penetrated the mucous membranes, frontal sinuses or cavities, their removal is more difficult. Major and irreversible damage may be done by the larvae.

The biologies and medical importance of the principal types of flies causing facultative and obligatory myiasis in man are outlined below.

CLASSIFICATION

The flies in this chapter are contained in three main families, the Calliphoridae, the Sarcophagidae and the Cuterebridae. The family Calliphoridae can be conveniently divided into a group containing the non-metallic flies such as the Congo floor-maggot fly (*Auchmeromyia senegalensis* (= *luteola*)), the tumbu fly (*Cordylobia anthropophaga*) and the metallic calliphorids. Well-known examples of the metallic group are the blowflies, comprising the bluebottles (*Calliphora*), the greenbottles (*Lucilia*), the New World screw-worm (*Cochliomyia hominivorax*) and the Old World screw-worm (*Chrysomya bezziana*).

THE NON-METALLIC CALLIPHORIDS
Cordylobia anthropophaga

External morphology

This species is known as the tumbu or mango fly and is found only in Africa, occurring from Ethiopia in the north through West and East Africa to Natal and Transvaal in the south.

Adults are robust, relatively big flies, about 9–12 mm long, dull yellowish to light brown in colour, but with two dark grey and poorly defined dorsal longitudinal thoracic stripes (Fig. 10.1). There are four visible abdominal segments which are more or less equal in length (compare *Auchmeromyia senegalensis* in which the second abdominal segment is markedly longer than the others). The wings are slightly brownish.

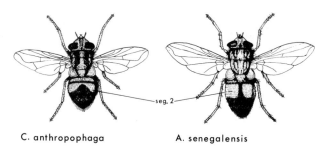

C. anthropophaga   A. senegalensis

Fig. 10.1 Adults of the tumbu fly (*Cordylobia anthropophaga*) and the Congo floor-maggot fly (*Auchmeromyia senegalensis*) showing differences in length of 2nd abdominal segment.

Life-cycle

Females lay up to 100–300 eggs in batches on dry soil and sand in shady places, especially when contaminated with the urine or excreta of man, rodents, dogs or monkeys. Females also oviposit on underclothes or soiled nappies (diapers) of babies placed on the ground to dry. The eggs, which are white and banana-shaped, hatch after about 1–2 days. Larvae attach themselves to a suitable host either directly, or attach themselves temporarily to washed clothing placed on the ground to dry, and so get transferred to man if the clothing is not ironed before wearing. Once on a host, powerful hook-like mouthparts enable a larva to bury itself completely except for its posterior spiracles situated at the tip of the abdomen, which remain in contact with the air. Newly emerged larvae can live as long as 9–15 days on the ground in the absence of a suitable host before they die.

The minute 1st-instar larvae are typically maggot-shaped, the 2nd-instar larvae are club-shaped, while the 3rd- and final instar larvae are rather fat, broadly oval-shaped, yellowish-white maggots, about 11–15 mm long. They are covered with numerous spicules which are often, but not always, grouped into three or more transverse rows per segment (Fig. 10.2). After 10–12 days mature larvae wriggle out of the boil-like swellings and fall to the ground where they bury themselves and turn into puparia. Adult flies emerge some 10 days later and readily enter houses, especially mud huts, where they may lay their eggs on the mud floors especially if children have urinated on them.

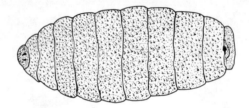

Fig. 10.2   Final instar larva of the tumbu fly (*Cordylobia anthropophaga*).

Medical importance

Larvae of *Cordylobia* cause boil-like (furuncular) swellings on almost any part of the body. Although these swellings may become sore and inflamed, and even quite hard and exude serous fluids, they do not usually contain pus. The standard method of extracting a larva is to cover the small hole in the swelling with medicinal liquid paraffin. This prevents the larva from breathing through its posterior spiracles with the result that it wriggles a little further out of the swelling to protrude the spiracles. In so doing it lubricates the pocket in the skin, and the larva can then usually be extracted by gently pressing around the swelling.

Infections are prevented by wearing shoes and ensuring that clothes, bed linen and towels are not spread on the ground to dry.

Dogs are commonly infected with tumbu larvae.

Auchmeromyia senegalensis

External morphology

These flies, commonly known as Congo floor-maggot flies, although not strictly speaking producing myiasis, are described here because the adults are often confused with those of *Cordylobia anthropophaga*. They occur throughout Africa south of the Sahara and also in the Cape Verde islands.

Adults are very similar to *C. anthropophaga* but are distinguished by the second abdominal segment being about twice as long as any of the others (see Fig. 10.1); whereas in the tumbu fly all segments are about equal in length.

Life-cycle and medical importance

Eggs are laid in batches of about 50 on the dry sandy floors of mud huts. They hatch after 1–3 days and the larvae hide away in cracks and crevices in the hut floor, especially under beds and sleeping mats. At night the larvae crawl out from these daytime refuges and take blood-meals from sleeping people within the hut. After taking a full blood-meal the now pinkish larvae return to their hiding places. Larvae may feed about 4–5 times a week, but can withstand starvation for long periods in the absence of suitable hosts. There are three larval instars each requiring at least two blood-meals. Under optimum conditions larval development is completed within 3–4 weeks, but this period may be prolonged to as long as 3 months if the larvae fail to obtain regular feeds. The fully developed 3rd-instar larvae, unlike those of *Cordylobia anthropophaga*, are not covered with spicules (Fig. 10.3). Larvae cannot climb, and therefore people will not be attacked if they sleep on beds raised from the floors by only short legs. Mature

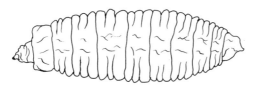

Fig. 10.3 Final instar larva of the Congo floor-maggot fly (*Auchmeromyia senegalensis.*

larvae pupate in cracks or directly on the surface of the mud floor of huts. Adults emerge from the puparia after about 9–16 days.

The Congo floor-maggot used to be quite common in certain parts of Africa, but due to the changes in life-style of most Africans it is becoming increasingly rare, and these days is not much of a problem.

THE METALLIC CALLIPHORIDS

New World screw-worms

The New World screw-worm, *Cochliomyia hominivorax*, occurs sporadically in southwestern USA down through Mexico to Argentina.

External morphology

Adult flies are 8–10 mm long, metallic green to bluish-green in colour and have three distinct dark longitudinal stripes on the dorsal surface of the thorax (Fig. 10.4). The dorsal bristles on the

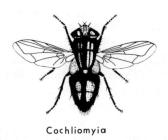

Cochliomyia

Fig. 10.4 Adult of New World screw-worm (*Cochliomyia*).

thorax, like those of *Chrysomya*, are poorly developed, thus distinguishing screw-worm flies from *Lucilia* and *Calliphora* which have well developed bristles. Examination under a microscope shows that the squama of the wing is covered with fine hairs on the dorsal surface (Fig. 10.5a), thus differing from *Lucilia* adults which have the squama without hairs.

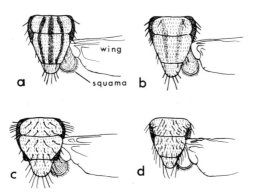

Fig. 10.5 Thoraces and bases of right wings showing presence or absence of well developed thoracic dorsal bristles, and fine hairs on squama at base of wings. (a) *Cochliomyia*, note three dark thoracic stripes; (b) *Chrysomya*, note two thoracic stripes; (c) *Calliphora*, note well developed thoracic bristles and hairy squama; (d) *Lucilia*, note well developed thoracic hairs and hairless squama.

Life-cycle

Females of *C. hominivorax* lay batches of 10–400 eggs on the edges of 2- to 10-day-old wounds, scabs, sores, scratches or pimples, also on dried blood clots and on diseased and even healthy mucous membranes such as nasal passages, the mouth and vagina. In new-born babies eggs are laid in the umbilicus. Eggs hatch within 11–22 hours and the active larvae bury deeply into the living tissues and feed gregariously. There are three larval instars and the 3rd-instar larvae, which are formed after 2–3 days, are

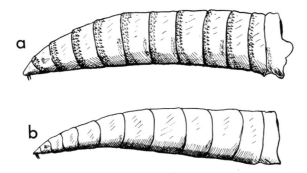

Fig. 10.6 Final instar larvae. (a) *Cochliomyia hominivorax*; (b) *Lucilia* species (*Calliphora* larvae are almost identical).

about 15–17 mm long and typically maggot-shaped. They are distinguished from housefly maggots by the presence of distinct bands of spicules encircling the anterior margins of all body segments (Fig. 10.6a). Larvae tend to penetrate deeply into tissues so that infections near the eyes, nose and mouth can cause considerable destruction of these areas, often accompanied by putrid smelling discharges and ulcerations.

After 4–8 days the larvae reach maturity and wriggle out of the wounds or passages they have excavated by devouring living tissue and drop to the ground, where they bury in the soil and pupate. In warm weather the puparial stage lasts about 7–10 days, but in cooler weather may be prolonged for many weeks or even months. Under optimum conditions the life-cycle from egg to egg is about 24 days.

Old World screw-worms

The genus *Chrysomya* contains many species and is common in the tropics. About ten species are known to cause myiasis in man, but only *Chrysomya bezziana* is important because its larvae are obligatory parasites of living tissues. Larvae of the other species are not obligatory parasites and often develop in carrion and decomposing matter. *C. bezziana* occurs throughout tropical Africa and most of Asia, ranging from India to the Philippines, Celebes, New Guinea and China, but the fly is absent from Australia.

External morphology

Adults are very similar to *Cochliomyia*, but there are only two indistinct longitudinal thoracic stripes (see Fig. 10.5b). Larvae are also very similar to those of *Cochliomyia*, although there are minor morphological differences. In practice separation is easy: screw-worms of the Americas belong to the genus *Cochliomyia* while those in the Old World belong to the genus *Chrysomya*.

Life-cycle

The life-cycle is very similar to that of *Cochliomyia hominivorax*. About 150–500 eggs are deposited in wounds, several days old, open sores, scabs, ulcers, gums, scratches or on mucous membranes, especially those contaminated with discharges. Newly emerged larvae burrow through the skin to the underlying tissues where they commonly remain congregated together. Larvae complete their development in 5–6 days and then wriggle out of the wounds and drop to the ground, where they bury themselves and pupate. The puparial period lasts about 7–9 days in warm weather, but is prolonged to several weeks or even months during cold weather. The life-cycle from egg to egg under ideal conditions is about 22 days.

Adults of both the New and Old World screw-worms are frequently found feeding on decomposing corpses, decaying matter, excreta and flowers.

Medical importance of screw-worms

Larvae of both *Chrysomya bezziana* and *Cochliomyia hominivorax* are obligatory parasites of living tissues and cause human myiasis, which can be very severe resulting in considerable damage and disfigurement, especially if the face is attacked. When larvae invade natural orifices, such as the nose, mouth, eyes or vagina, they can cause excruciating pain and misery. In one patient suffering from a nasal infection 385 larvae of *C. hominivorax* were removed over a 9-day period! Larvae of both species may eat their way through the palate and as a result impair speech.

All myiasis cases should be treated immediately because the very rapid larval development can soon cause permanent damage.

C. bezziana seems to cause more cases of myiasis in people in India and other parts of Asia than it does in Africa. *Chrysomya* adults commonly visit faeces, so are potential vectors of several pathogens.

Both screw-worm species cause myiasis in cattle, horses, goats, sheep and other animals. In the USA prior to 1958 the livestock industry lost an estimated 120 million dollars a year due to *C. hominivorax*.

The greenbottles (*Lucilia*)

External morphology

There are several species of greenbottles within the genus *Lucilia* and although the genus has a world-wide distribution most species occur in northern temperate regions. They are mostly metallic or coppery green in colour, usually a little smaller (about 10 mm long) and a little less bristly than species of *Calliphora* (bluebottles). As in *Calliphora*, prominent bristles are present on the dorsal surface of the thorax (see Fig. 10.5d), but whereas the squama of the wing is hairy dorsally in bluebottles it is without hairs in *Lucilia* (see Fig. 10.5d). *Lucilia sericata* is the commonest species, occurring in the Americas, Europe, Asia, Africa, Australia and in most other areas of the world. Another common species, *L. cuprina*, occurs mainly in Africa, Asia and Australia.

Life-cycle

Female greenbottles normally lay their eggs on meat, fish, carrion and decaying or decomposing carcasses, but they will also oviposit on or near festering and foul-smelling wounds of man and animals, and also on excreta and decaying vegetable matter. Eggs hatch within 8-12 hours. Larvae are typically maggot-shaped (see Fig. 10.6b). They do not bear spicules as do larvae of the screw-worms, and therefore resemble larvae of the common housefly, from which they can be separated by the form of the posterior spiracles which are not D-shaped.

The larval period lasts about 4-8 days. Mature larvae bury in loose soil and pupate, the puparial period lasting about 6-14 days.

Adult flies frequently visit carrion, excreta, general refuse, decaying material, sores and wounds. They are particularly common around unhygienic places and situations where meat or decaying animals are present. They are nearly always abundant near slaughterhouses and piggeries. They commonly fly into houses, where they are particularly troublesome because of their noisy buzzing flights. The most common species infesting wounds of humans are *Lucilia sericata* and *L. cuprina*.

The bluebottles (*Calliphora*)

External morphology

These flies are usually known as bluebottles, they belong to the genus *Calliphora*. Although *Calliphora* has a world-wide distribution bluebottles are more common in the northern temperate regions than in the tropical or southern temperate regions.

Adults are robust flies, mostly dull metallic-bluish or bluish-black in colour and 8–14 mm long. As in *Lucilia* there are well developed bristles on the thorax (see Fig. 10.5c), but the squama of the wing is hairy on the dorsal surface (see Fig. 10.5c) whereas in *Lucilia* it lacks hairs. The abdomen is rather more shiny than the thorax.

Life-cycle

Larvae look very similar to those of *Lucilia*, and the life-cycle is also very similar to that described for *Lucilia*.

Medical importance of greenbottles and bluebottles

The dirty habit of blowflies (greenbottles and bluebottles) of alighting and feeding on excreta, decaying material and virtually all common foods of man make them potential mechanical vectors of a number of pathogens. It has been suggested that *Lucilia sericata* may aid the transmission of poliomyelitis, transfer of the virus occurring when flies feed on carrion and then wounds. However, their medical importance is usually associated with facultative myiasis.

Larvae of both *Lucilia* and *Calliphora* have been found in many parts of the world developing in foul-smelling wounds and ulcerations, especially those producing pus. They have also been recorded in hospitals underneath the bandages and dressings of patients, especially when these have become contaminated with blood and pus. Such infections do not usually cause any serious damage or harm since the larvae feed mainly on pus and dead tissues. In fact until comparatively recently they were sometimes used to cleanse septic wounds, and help prevent osteomyelitis. Very occasionally maggots which have infected wounds invade healthy tissues, and even more rarely infections with these maggots have caused a hand or leg to be amputated.

Occasionally intestinal myiasis is reported. This is usually caused by eating uncooked food contaminated with larvae of *Lucilia* or *Calliphora*, but usually the larvae are killed within the human alimentary canal and no serious harm is done. As emphasised previously (p. 155) there is no obligatory intestinal myiasis in man.

Control of greenbottles and bluebottles

The principal breeding places of greenbottles and bluebottles are
domestic refuse, rubbish tips, dustbins, offal and other wastes of
slaughterhouses, and meat packing factories. Larvae also occur in
foods such as meat and fish left out in the sun to dry. Any
methods which reduce the accumulation of these potential breeding sites are welcome. Dustbins and garbage cans should have
tight-fitting lids and be emptied once or twice a week. The outside of such bins and both sides of the lid can be sprayed with 5
per cent DDT or 0·5 per cent HCH every 7–10 days, and the
adjacent walls and fences sprayed every 2 weeks. This will deter
flies from ovipositing in these sites.

The reader is referred to Chapter 9 for control measures
against houseflies and related flies as many are applicable to
the *Calliphoridae*.

SARCOPHAGIDAE

Only the genera *Sarcophaga* and *Wohlfahrtia*, both of which
have several species, are of any medical importance. They cause
myiasis, and possibly act as mechanical vectors of pathogens.
They are sometimes called fleshflies. They have a world-wide
distribution.

Sarcophaga

External morphology

These are large and hairy non-metallic flies, about 10–15 mm
long, and usually greyish in colour. They have three prominent
black longitudinal dorsal stripes on the thorax. The abdomen is
sometimes distinctly, but other times indistinctly, marked with
squarish dark patches on a grey background giving it a chequer-
board (chess-board) appearance (Fig. 10.7).

Life-cycle and medical importance

Adults do not lay eggs but deposit 1st-instar larvae, as do tsetse
flies and *Wohlfahrtia*. The larvae are deposited in batches of 20–

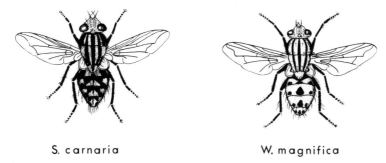

S. carnaria   W. magnifica

Fig. 10.7 Adults of *Sarcophaga carnaria* and *Wohlfahrtia magnifica* showing differences in abdominal markings.

40, usually on decaying carcasses, rotting food and human and animal excreta, but sometimes in wounds. They are primarily scavengers. Larvae are typically maggot-shaped. They are distinguised from larvae of the Calliphoridae because the posterior spiracles are situated in a deep pit (Fig. 10.8), and are thus difficult to see, and also because they have bands of spicules on the body. Larvae of *Sarcophaga* are not easily distinguished from those of *Wohlfahrtia*.

Larval development is rapid, lasting in hot weather in the presence of nutritious food supply only 3–4 days, at the end of which time they bury in the soil and pupate. The puparial stage lasts about 7–12 days.

Although larvae are normally deposited in carrion they very occasionally occur in wounds, but usually they cause little damage as they feed mainly on necrotic tissues. They have more commonly been incriminated with accidental intestinal myiasis, causing considerable discomfort and pain before the larvae are passed out with the faeces. The most common species is *Sarcophaga haemorrhoidalis*, which is widely distributed in the Americas, Europe, Africa and Asia. Because adults frequent festering wounds, excreta and decaying animal matter they may be mechanical vectors of various pathogens.

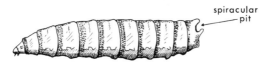

spiracular pit

Fig. 10.8 Larva of *Sarcophaga carnaria* showing deep pit in which posterior spiracles are located. (*Wohlfahrtia* larvae are almost identical).

Wohlfahrtia

External morphology

These are hairy flies about as large, or a little larger, than blue-bottles. They are greyish and like *Sarcophaga* have three distinct black lines on the dorsal surface of the thorax. The dark markings on the abdomen, however, are not in the form of a chess-board pattern as in *Sarcophaga* species, but are usually present as roundish lateral spots and triangular-shaped dark markings along the midline (see Fig. 10.7). There is, however, considerable variation and sometimes the dark marks are so large as to be more or less confluent, making the abdomen appear mainly black.

Life-cycle and medical importance

As with *Sarcophaga* and tsetse flies, adults of *Wohlfahrtia* deposit larvae not eggs. These are deposited in batches of 50–70 in scratches, wounds, sores and ulcerations on man and animals. They are sometimes deposited in the ear, nose or eyes, and in these sites they can cause considerable pain and extensive damage, and may even rarely cause death. A great number of domestic pets and farmyard animals are also attacked by the larvae. The North American species, W. *vigil*, will also deposit its larvae on unbroken skin if it is soft and tender, such as in babies and very young children, who are, therefore, more commonly attacked than adults. *Wohlfahrtia* larvae have bands of spicules, and the spiracles are situated in a deep pit (see Fig. 10.8). They are very similar in appearance to those of *Sarcophaga*. Larval development takes 5–10 days, mature larvae drop to the ground and bury amongst loose soil and then pupate. Adults emerge from the puparia after 8–12 days.

Wohlfahrtia larvae remain in the dermal tissues, and therefore do not cause such extensive damage and discomfort as the screw-worms, which bury deeper into the tissues.

CUTEREBRIDAE

Dermatobia hominis is the only species of medical importance in the family, it causes myiasis. It is found in Central and South

America, from Mexico down to northern Argentina. It also occurs in Trinidad but is apparently absent from all other West Indian islands.

Dermatobia hominis

External morphology

These flies are sometimes known as human botflies, or by a variety of local names such as 'bernefly' and 'ver macaque'.

Adults are a little larger (12–18 mm) than bluebottles (*Calliphora*) but have a similar dark-blue metallic-coloured abdomen, dark bluish-grey thorax and a mainly yellowish head. They are readily separated from all other flies of medical importance by the mask-like flap that hangs down from the head and hides the vestigial mouthparts (Fig. 10.9).

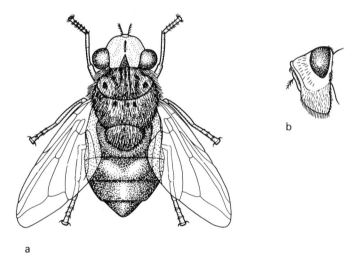

a
b

Fig. 10.9 *Dermatobia hominis*. (a) Dorsal view of adult; (b) lateral view of head showing flap-like mask.

Life-cycle

The fly occurs primarily in lowland forests, being especially common along woodland paths and at the margins of forest and scrub areas. These flies have an interesting and remarkable life-history. Females glue 6–30 eggs to the body of other arthropods, such as ticks or various Diptera, most of which are blood-sucking flies. The most commonly involved insects are day-biting mosquitoes, especially those belonging to the genus *Psorophora*, but stableflies (*Stomoxys calcitrans*) often have eggs stuck to their bodies too.

Embryos within the attached eggs mature into 1st-instar larvae within 4–9 days. They do not hatch, however, until the insects carrying the eggs settle on man or some other warm-blooded animal, or even birds, to take a blood-meal or, as in the case of houseflies, feed on sweat. The larvae then emerge from the eggs, which remain attached to the insect carrier, and drop on to the host's skin. Here, within 5–15 minutes, the larvae manage to penetrate the skin and bury into the subcutaneous tissues. Each larva produces a boil-like swelling which has an opening through which the larva breathes.

The 1st-instar larvae are 1–1·5 mm long, more or less cylindrical in shape (Fig. 10.10a), and have the anterior half of the body covered with numerous spines of two different sizes. The 2nd-instar larvae are a completely different shape, being enlarged anteriorly but with the posterior half of the body distinctly narrow, giving the appearance of a bottle with a long neck. Relatively large thorn-like spines encircle the middle segments (Fig. 10.10b). The 3rd- and final instar larvae are about 18–25 mm long, more or less oval and have relatively small spines on the anterior segments (Fig. 10.10c). A pair of very distinct flower-like spiracles are present anteriorly, while less conspicuous slit-like spiracles are situated in a small concavity of the last abdominal segment.

Larval development is completed in a small pocket excavated

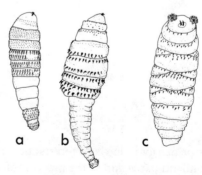

a   b   c

Fig. 10.10 *Dermatobia hominis* larvae. (a) 1st-instar; (b) 2nd-instar; (c) 3rd-instar.

in the subdermal layer of the host, and last about 4–18 weeks. Mature larvae wriggle out of the skin and drop to the ground where they pupate just under the surface of the soil. Adult flies emerge from the puparia after about 4–10 weeks, but are rarely seen.

Medical importance

Larvae of *Dermatobia hominis* invade the subcutaneous tissues of man on various parts of his body, including the head, arms, abdomen, buttocks, thighs, scrotum and axillae. They produce boil-like swellings which suppurate and this may attract other myiasis-producing flies to the host. They can cause a lot of discomfort and considerable pain. Because of the long duration of the larval life (up to 18 weeks) infected persons may be encountered in almost any part of the world.

Treatment consists of the surgical removal of the larvae under sterile conditions, frequently a local anaesthetic is necessary.

OTHER MYIASIS-PRODUCING FLIES

Several other species of flies commonly cause myiasis in livestock, and occasionally man becomes infected. People most likely to become infected are those working closely with the flies' natural hosts. There are for example flies that cause myiasis in sheep and goats, cattle and horses, and their larvae sometimes attack man.

Chapter 11
Fleas

There are possibly some 3000 species and subspecies of fleas, belonging to about 200 genera, but only relatively few are important pests of man. About 94 per cent of known species bite mammals and the remainder are parasites of birds. Fleas are found throughout most of the world, but many species and genera have a more restricted distribution, for example the genus *Xenopsylla*, which contains important plague vectors, is confined to the tropics and subtropics.

Medically the most important fleas are *Xenopsylla* species, such as *X. cheopis*, which is a vector of plague (*Yersinia pestis*), and flea-borne endemic typhus (*Rickettsia mooseri*). Some fleas, such as *Ctenocephalides* species, are intermediate hosts of cestodes (*Dipylidium caninum*, ?*Hymenolepis nana*, *H. diminuta*). Fleas may also be vectors of tularaemia (*Pasteurella tularensis*), while the chigoe or jigger flea (*Tunga penetrans*) burrows into the feet of man.

EXTERNAL MORPHOLOGY

Adults are relatively small (1-4 mm), and more or less oval insects, compressed laterally and varying in colour from light to dark brown. Wings are absent, but there are three pairs of powerful and well developed legs, the hind pair of which are specialised for jumping. The legs, and also much of the body, are covered with bristles and small spines.

The head is roughly triangular in shape, bears a pair of conspicuous black eyes (a few species are eyeless), and short three-segmented more or less club-shaped antennae which lie in depressions behind the eyes. The mouthparts point downwards. In some species a row of coarse, well developed and tooth-like spines, collectively known as the genal comb or genal ctenidium, is present along the bottom margin of the head capsule (Figs 11.1 and 11.2).

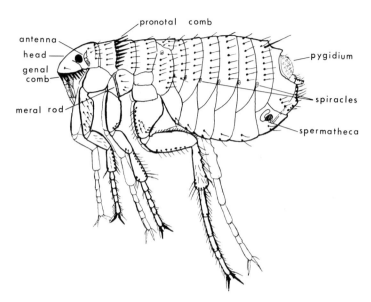

Fig. 11.1 Lateral view of adult flea showing position of combs and meral rod.

The thorax has three distinct segments, the pro-, meso- and metathorax. The posterior margin of the pronotum may bear a row of teeth-like coarse spines forming the pronotal comb or pronotal ctenidium (Fig. 11.1). Some genera of fleas lack both the pronotal and genal combs and are referred to as combless fleas (Fig. 11.2), whereas in some other genera both combs are present (Fig. 11.2). A sternite called the mesosternum (mesopleuron) is located above the middle pair of legs. In several genera, including *Xenopsylla*, which contains important plague vectors, this sternite is clearly divided into two parts by a thick vertical rod-like structure termed the meral rod or mesopleural suture. The presence of a meral rod, combined with the absence of both genal and pronotal combs, indicates the genus *Xenopsylla* (Fig. 11.2). However, it must be stressed that the presence of a meral rod by itself does not identify fleas as species of *Xenopsylla*, because several other genera which have combs also have a meral rod.

Male fleas are identified by the upturned appearance of the abdomen. In the female the tip of the abdomen is more rounded than in the male, and lying internally in about the position of the 6th–8th abdominal segments is a distinct brownish spermatheca

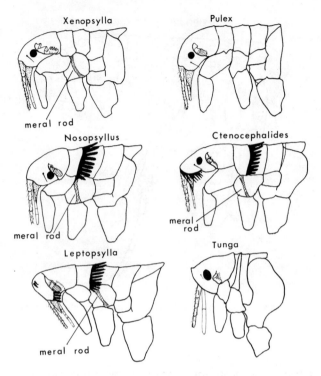

Fig. 11.2 Diagram of the head and first three thoracic segments of adult fleas belonging to six important genera.

(Fig. 11.1). It is not always important to separate the sexes as both take blood-meals and can be vectors of disease.

THE ALIMENTARY CANAL OF ADULT FLEAS

For a better understanding of the role fleas have in the transmission of plague it is necessary to describe the alimentary canal and the method of blood-feeding.

During feeding saliva is injected and the host's blood is sucked up through the spindle-shaped pharynx and thin oesophagus into the bulbous proventriculus (Fig. 11.3). This is provided internally with numerous backwardly projecting stiff spines which when pressed together prevent the regurgitation of the blood-meal into the oesophagus (Fig. 11.3). (The proventriculus is important in the mechanism of plague transmission.) Finally, the

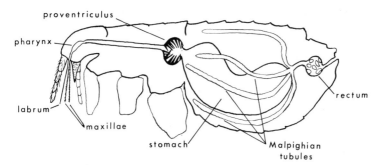

Fig. 11.3 Diagrammatic representation of the alimentary canal of an adult flea showing backwardly projecting spines in proventriculus.

blood-meal enters a relatively large stomach (mid gut) where it is digested. The distal end of the stomach is connected to the hind gut, the junction being easily identified by the four Malpighian tubules. The hind gut is continuous with a small dilated rectum which has prominent rectal papillae. These papillae extract water from the faeces, so that it passes out through the anus in an almost dry state.

LIFE-CYCLE

Both sexes of fleas take blood-meals and are therefore equally important as vectors of disease. The present account is a generalised description of the life-cycle of fleas which may occur on man or animals, such as dogs, cats and commensal rats. The life-cycle of the chigoe (*Tunga penetrans*) is described separately.

A female flea which is ready to oviposit may leave the host to deposit her eggs in debris which accumulates in the host's dwelling place, such as rodent burrows or nests. With species which occur on man or his domestic pets, such as cats and dogs, females often lay their eggs in or near cracks and crevices on the floor or amongst dust, dirt and debris. Sometimes, however, eggs are laid while the flea is still on the host and these usually, but not always, fall to the ground. The eggs are very small, oval, white or yellowish and lack any pattern. They are thinly coated with a sticky substance which usually results in them becoming covered with dirt and debris. Adult fleas may live for up to 6-12 months, or possibly 2 years or more, and during this time a female may lay 300-1000 eggs, mostly in small batches of about 3-18 a day.

Eggs hatch within about 2–14 days depending on the species of
flea, temperature and also humidity. A minute legless larva
emerges from the egg (Fig. 11.4). It has a small blackish head
with a very small pair of antennae, followed by 13 pale-brown,
distinct and more or less similar segments. Each segment bears a
circle of setae near the posterior border. The last segment ends
in a pair of finger-like ventral processes termed the anal struts.
The presence of these struts, combined with the setae on the
body, distinguish larval fleas from all other types of insects of
medical importance.

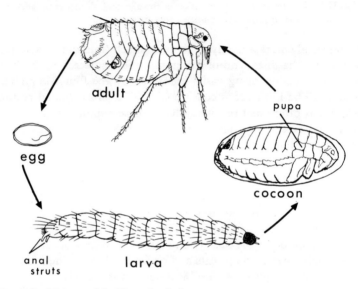

Fig. 11.4   Diagram of the life-cycle of a flea.

Larvae are very active. They avoid light and seek shelter in
cracks and crevices and amongst debris on floors of houses, or at
the bottom of nests and animal burrows. Sometimes, however,
larvae are found amongst the fur of animals, and even on people
who have unclean habits and dirt-laden clothes, and occasionally
in beds. Larvae feed on almost any organic debris including the
host's faeces, and partly digested blood evacuated from the alimentary canal of adult fleas; in a few species feeding on expelled
blood seems to be a nutritional requirement for larval development. In some species larvae are scavengers and feed on small
dead insects or dead adult fleas of their own kind. There are

usually three larval instars, but in some species there are only two instars. The larval period may last as little as 10–21 days, but this varies greatly according to species, and may be prolonged more than 200 days by unfavourable conditions such as limited food supply and low temperatures. Mature larvae are 4–10 mm long. Unlike adult fleas, larvae cannot tolerate large extremes in relative humidity and they die if humidities are either too low or too high.

At the end of the larval period the larva spins a whitish cocoon from silk produced by the larval salivary glands. Because of its sticky nature it soon becomes covered with fine particles of dust, organic debris and sand picked up from the floor of the host's home. Cocoons camouflaged in this way are very difficult to distinguish from their surroundings. About 2–3 days after having spun a cocoon around itself the larva pupates within the cocoon. Adults emerge from the pupa after about 7–14 days, but this period depends on the ambient temperature. After having emerged from the pupa the adult flea requires a stimulus, usually vibrations, such as caused by the movements of the host within its home, burrow or nest, before it escapes from the cocoon. If, however, animal shelters or houses are vacated, then adult fleas fail to escape from their cocoons until their dwelling places are reoccupied. In some species, carbon dioxide emitted from hosts or a seasonal increase in humidity stimulates emergence. Adults may remain alive in their cocoons for about 1 year. This explains why people moving into buildings which have been vacated for many months may be suddenly attacked by large numbers of very bloodthirsty fleas, these being newly emerged adults seeking their first blood-meal.

The life-cycle from egg to adult emergence may be as short as 2–3 weeks for certain species under optimum conditions, but frequently the life-cycle is considerably longer, such as 20 months or more.

Fleas avoid light and are therefore usually found sheltering amongst the hairs or feathers of animals, or on man under his clothing or in his bed. If given the opportunity many species of fleas feed several times during the day or night on their hosts. While feeding, fleas eject faeces composed at first of semi-digested blood of the previous meal and then excess blood taken in during the act of feeding. This mixture of partially digested and virtually undigested blood often marks clothing and bed linen of people heavily infected with fleas.

Although most species of fleas have one or two favourite species of hosts, they are not entirely host-specific, for example, cat and dog fleas (*Ctenocephalides felis* and *C. canis*) will readily feed on man, especially in the absence of their normal hosts. Human fleas (*Pulex irritans*) feed on pigs, and rat fleas of the genus *Xenopsylla* will attack man in the absence of rats. Most fleas will in fact bite other hosts in their immediate vicinity when their normal hosts are absent or scarce. However, although feeding on less acceptable hosts keeps fleas alive, their fertility can be seriously reduced by continued feeding on such hosts. Fleas rapidly abandon dead hosts to seek out new ones, behaviour which is of profound epidemiological importance in plague transmission. Fleas can withstand both considerable desiccation and prolonged periods of starvation, for example 6 months or more when no suitable hosts are present. On their host, fleas move either by rapidly crawling or by jumping, but off the host they tend to jump more than crawl in their search for new hosts. Fleas can jump about 20 cm vertically and 30 cm or more horizontally. (Such remarkable feats are achieved through a rubber-like protein called resilin, which is very elastic and can become highly compressed; rapid expansion of the uncompressed state gives the power for jumping.)

MEDICAL IMPORTANCE

Flea nuisance

Although certain species of fleas may be important vectors of disease, the most widespread complaint about them concerns the annoyance caused by their bites, which in some people lead to considerable discomfort and irritation. The three most widespread and common nuisance fleas are the cat and dog fleas, *Ctenocephalides felis* and *C. canis*, and to a lesser extent the so-called human flea, *Pulex irritans*. In some areas other species such as the European chicken flea (*Ceratophyllus gallinae*) and the Western chicken flea (*C. niger*) may be of local importance.

Fleas frequently bite people on the ankles and legs, but at night a sleeping person is bitten on other parts of the body. In many people the bite is felt almost immediately, but irritation usually becomes worse some time after biting. In sensitised people intense itching may result. Because fleas are difficult to catch this tends to increase the annoyance they cause, and people attacked by fleas frequently spend sleepless nights alternately scratching themselves and trying to catch the fleas. There is evidence that children under 10 years generally experience greater discomfort than older people.

Plague

Plague is caused by *Yersinia pestis* and is primarily a disease of wild animals, especially rodents, not man. Over 220 rodent species have been shown to harbour plague bacilli. The cycle of transmission of plague between wild rodents, such as gerbils, marmots, voles, chipmunks and ground squirrels, is termed sylvatic, campestral, rural or endemic plague. Many different species of fleas bite these rodents and maintain plague transmission amongst them. When people such as fur trappers and hunters handle these wild animals there is the risk that they will get bitten by rodent fleas and become infected with plague.

An important form of plague is urban plague. This describes the situation when plague circulating amongst the wild rodent population has been transmitted to commensal rats, and is maintained in the rat population by fleas such as *Xenopsylla cheopis* (Europe, Asia, Africa and the Americas), *X. astia* (South-east Asia) and *X. brasiliensis* (Africa, South America and India). When rats are living in close association with man, such as rat-infested slums, fleas normally feeding on rats may turn their attention to man. This is most likely to happen when rats are infected with plague and as a result rapidly develop an acute and fatal septicaemia. On death of the rats the infected fleas leave their more normal hosts and feed on man. In this way plague is spread by rat fleas to the human population. The most important vector species is *X. cheopis*, but some 29 other species of fleas have been found to transmit plague, including *Xenopsylla astia*, *X. brasiliensis*; and more rarely *Nosopsyllus fasciatus* and *Leptopsylla aethiopica*, species which are normally reluctant to bite man, and also the cat and dog fleas. In addition to man becoming infected by the bite of fleas which have previously fed on infected rats, the disease can also be spread from man to man by fleas, such as *Xenopsylla* species and *Pulex irritans*, feeding on a plague victim then on another person. This latter method, however, appears to play a minor role in the transmission of plague.

It is important to understand the methods by which fleas

transmit plague. Plague bacilli sucked up with the blood-meals of male and female fleas are passed to the stomach where they undergo so great a multiplication that they extend forwards to invade the proventriculus. In some species, especially those of the genus *Xenopsylla*, further multiplication in the proventriculus may result in it becoming partially, or more or less completely, blocked. This prevents the proventriculus from functioning normally and results in fleas regurgitating some of the blood-meal during later feeds. Thus, plague bacilli obtained from a previous feed are passed down the flea's mouthparts into the host. In the case of completely blocked fleas, blood is sucked up with considerable difficulty about as far as the proventriculus, where it mixes with the bacilli and is then regurgitated back into the new host. Blocked fleas soon become starved and repeatedly bite in attempts to get a blood-meal, and are therefore potentially very dangerous. Even if there is no blockage of the alimentary canal, plague transmission can nevertheless occur by direct contamination from the flea's mouthparts.

Another, but less important, method of infection is by the flea's faeces being rubbed into abrasions in the skin or coming into contact with mucous membranes. Plague bacilli can remain infective in flea faeces for as long as 3 years. Occasionally the tonsils become infected with plague bacilli due to crushing infected fleas between the teeth.

In pneumonic plague the bacilli occur in enormous numbers in the sputum. This form of plague is highly contagious due to the ease by which bacilli are transmitted from patients to others by coughing, and the inhalation of droplets; insects are not involved in the spread of pneumonic plague.

Flea-borne endemic typhus

Flea-borne or murine typhus is caused by *Rickettsia mooseri* which is ingested by the flea with its blood-meal. Within the gut the rickettsiae multiply, but unlike plague bacilli they do not cause any blockage of the proventriculus or stomach. Infection is caused by infected faeces being rubbed into abrasions or coming into contact with delicate mucous membranes, and also by the release of rickettsiae from crushed fleas. Faeces may remain infective under ideal conditions for as long as 4–9 years. Murine typhus is essentially a disease of rodents, particularly rats and especially *Rattus rattus* and *R. norvegicus*. It is spread amongst rats and other rodents by *Xenopsylla* species, especially *X. cheopis*, but also by *Nosopsyllus fasciatus*, *Leptopsylla segnis* and by a few ectoparasites which are not fleas, such as the rat louse *Polyplax spinulosa* (possibly also *Hoplopleura* spp.) and maybe by the tropical rat mite *Ornithonyssus bacoti*. Man becomes infected mainly through *Xenopsylla cheopis*, but occasionally *Nosopsyllus fasciatus*, *Ctenocephalides canis*, *C. felis* and *Pulex irritans* may be involved. *Leptopsylla segnis* does not attack man, but it is possible that murine typhus is sometimes spread to man by an aerosol of infective faeces of this species.

Cestodes

Dipylidium caninum is one of the more common tapeworms of dogs and cats and occasionally occurs in children, while *Hymenolepis diminuta* infects rats and mice and occasionally man. These tapeworms can be transmitted by fleas to both rodents and man. Eggs of these parasites are passed out with excreta of rats and domestic pets and may be swallowed by larval fleas feeding on excreta. Larval worms hatching from the ingested eggs penetrate the gut wall of the larval flea and pass across into the body cavity (coelom). They remain trapped within this space and pass on to the pupa and finally to the adult flea where they encapsulate and become cysticercoids (infective larvae). Animals can become infected by licking their coats during grooming and thus swallowing the infected adult fleas. Similarly, young children fondling and kissing dogs and cats can become infected with *D. caninum* by swallowing cat and dog fleas, or by being licked by dogs which have crushed infected fleas in their mouths thus liberating the infective cysticercoids. Adult rat fleas (*Xenopsylla*, *Nosopsyllus*) occasionally get mixed with food or drink and swallowed by man, who may then become infected with *Hymenolepis diminuta*.

Another tapeworm of man, *H. nana*, is spread through contaminated food or water, and possibly also by fleas but their role in transmission is unclear because a morphologically identical parasite, *H. fraterna* of rats and mice, has fleas, especially *Xenopsylla* species, as intermediate hosts. *H. nana* is known to be capable of developing in insects, and it is possible that fleas and rodents sometimes serve as intermediate hosts and reservoirs of infection, respectively.

Less important diseases

In addition to the above diseases and parasites spread by fleas these insects may play some small part in the transmission of *Pasteurella tularensis*, *Rickettsia conori* and *Coxiella burneti*. However, it should be stressed that their role as vectors of these pathogens is at the most minimal.

TUNGA PENETRANS

External morphology

Tunga penetrans is found in the tropics and subtropics, having a distribution stretching from Central and South America, the West Indies across Africa to Madagascar. It has occasionally been reported in persons in India returning from overseas, mainly Africa, but the flea is not indigenous to India or elsewhere in Asia. *Tunga penetrans* is sometimes referred to as the chigoe or

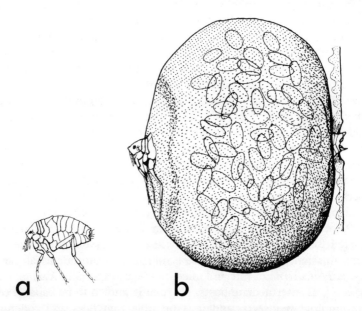

Fig. 11.5 Adults of *Tunga penetrans*. (a) Non-gravid (immature) female flea; (b) gravid female with enormously swollen abdomen full of eggs, embedded in skin of host. Tip of abdomen projects from host's skin to exterior.

jigger flea. *T. penetrans* does not transmit any disease to man but is a nuisance because females burrow into the skin.

Adults of both sexes are exceedingly small, only about 1 mm long (Fig. 11.5a). They have neither genal nor pronotal combs and are easily separated from other fleas of medical importance by their very compressed first three (thoracic) segments, and the paucity of spines and bristles on the body.

Life-cycle and medical importance

Eggs are dropped onto the floor of houses or on the ground outside. They hatch within about 3–4 days and the larvae inhabit dirty and dusty floors or dry sandy soils, especially in areas frequented by hosts of the adult fleas. Under favourable conditions larval development is completed within about 10–14 days, the pupal period lasts about 5–14 days, and the complete life-cycle can be as short as about 18 days.

Newly emerged adults are very agile and jump and crawl about on the ground until they locate a suitable host, which is usually a man or pig. Both sexes feed on blood, but whereas the male soon leaves the host after taking a blood-meal, the female, after being fertilised, burrows into the skin where it is soft such as between the toes or under toe-nails. Other areas of the foot, including the sole, may also be invaded. In people habitually sitting on the ground, such as beggars or infants, the buttocks may often be infected, and particularly heavy infestations have been recorded from leprosy patients. In heavily infected individuals the arms, especially the elbows, may also be attacked, and occasionally the females burrow into the soft skin around the genital region. Burrowing into the skin appears to be accomplished by the flea's sharp and well-developed mouthparts. The result is that the entire flea, with the exception of the tip of the abdomen bearing the anus, genital opening and large respiratory spiracles, becomes completely buried in the host's skin. In this embedded position she continues to feed. The area surrounding the embedded flea becomes very itchy and inflamed, and secondary infections may become established, resulting in ulcerations and accumulation of pus. While the blood-meal is being digested, the abdomen distends to a relatively enormous size and the flea attains both the shape and size (6 mm) of a small pea (Fig. 11.5b). This expansion is accomplished in some 8–10 days. Towards the end of this period of abdominal enlargement the ovaries are composed of thousands of minute eggs. Over the next 7–14 days about 150–200 eggs are passed out of the female genital opening, most of which eventually fall to the ground and hatch after about 3–4 days.

When the female fleas die they remain embedded within the host. This frequently causes inflammation and may, in addition, result in secondary infections, which if ignored can lead to loss of the toes, tetanus, or even gangrene. Male fleas cause no such trouble as they do not burrow into the skin.

These fleas are most common in people not wearing shoes, such as children. Because they are feeble jumpers, wearing shoes is a simple, but in some communities relatively costly, method of reducing the likelihood of flea infection.

Females embedded in the skin should be removed with fine needles under aseptic conditions, and wounds caused by their extraction sterilised and dressed. They are best removed within the first few days of their becoming established, as they are difficult to extract when they have greatly distended abdomens, containing numerous eggs, without rupturing them, and this increases the risk of infections.

Pigs, in addition to man, are often commonly invaded by *Tunga*, and they may provide a local reservoir of infection. Other animals such as cats, dogs and rats are also readily attacked.

CONTROL OF FLEAS

Cat and dog fleas (*Ctenocephalides felis* and *C. canis*) can most easily be detected by examination of the fur round the neck, or on the belly of the hosts. Proprietary insecticidal powders containing 1 per cent HCH, 2–5 per cent malathion, 2–5 per cent carbaryl (Sevin) or 1 per cent permethrin can be applied to the coat of an animal. A simple, but not always very efficient, procedure is to place a proprietary plastic collar impregnated with 20 per cent dichlorvos (DDVP) round the necks of dogs and cats. However, an important consideration is that most fleas are found away from the host, not on it. For example, it has been said that a typical colony of cat fleas consists of only about 25 adult fleas on the cat, but that on the floor and bedding there may be 500 adult fleas, 500 cocoons and as many as 3000 larvae and 1000 eggs. Clearly, control measures should not be restricted to the cat but applied to the total environment. Flea cocoons are not very susceptible to insecticides, consequently insecticidal treatments should be repeated about every 2 weeks for about 6 months. Beds, kennels, or other places where pests sleep, or spend much of their time, should be treated either with insecticidal powders or lightly sprayed with solutions containing 0·5 per cent HCH, 2 per cent malathion, 0·5 per cent diazinon or 2 per cent dichlorvos (DDVP), to kill both adult and larval fleas.

For more general control of fleas, powders of 5–10 per cent DDT, 1 per cent HCH or 0·5 per cent dieldrin can be liberally applied to floors of houses and runways of rodents. Insecticidal dusts can also be blown into rodent burrows. In many parts of the world, however, *Xenopsylla cheopis* and *Pulex irritans* have developed resistance to DDT, HCH and dieldrin. In such cases organophosphate or carbamate insecticides such as 2 per cent diazinon, 2 per cent fenthion (Baytex), 5 per cent malathion, 2 per cent fenitrothion (Sumithion), 5 per cent jodofenphos, or 3–5 per cent carbaryl (Sevin) can be used. In India *X. cheopis* has developed resistance to malathion, and trials in that country have shown carbaryl (Sevin) to be the most effective insecticide.

Insecticidal fogs or aerosols containing 2 per cent malathion or 2 per cent Ronnel have sometimes been used to fumigate houses harbouring fleas.

For the control of fleas in urban outbreaks of plague or murine typhus, extensive and well-organised insecticidal operations may be necessary. At the same time as insecticides are applied, rodenticides such as the anticoagulants, for example warfarin and fumarin, can be administered to kill the rodent population. However, if fast-acting 'one-dose' rodenticides such as zinc phosphide, sodium fluoracetate or strychnine or the more modern fast-acting anticoagulants like bromadiolone and chlorophacinone are used, then it is essential to apply these several days after insecticidal applications. Otherwise the rodents will be killed but not their fleas, which will then bite other mammals including man, and this may result in increasing disease transmission.

Insecticidal repellents such as dimethyl phthalate, diethyl-toluamide or benzyl benzoate may afford some personal protection against fleas.

Chapter 12
Lice

Blood-sucking lice of man are of three types and comprise the pubic or crab louse (*Pthirus pubis*), the body louse (*Pediculus humanus humanus = P. corporis*) and the head louse (*Pediculus humanus capitis*). Morphologically it is very difficult to separate head and body lice, in fact the two can interbreed in the laboratory, but there is little evidence that natural hybridisation occurs. Although treated here as subspecies, they are often given specific status. All three kinds of lice have a more or less world-wide distribution, but they are often more common in temperate areas.

Body lice are vectors of louse-borne typhus (*Rickettsia prowazeki*), trench fever (*Rochalimaea quintana*) and louse-borne relapsing fever (*Borrelia recurrentis*).

THE BODY LOUSE
(*PEDICULUS HUMANUS HUMANUS*)

External morphology

Adults are small, greyish and wingless insects, with a soft but rather leathery integument, and are flattened dorsoventrally (Fig. 12.1). Males measure about 2–3 mm and females about 3·0–4·5 mm. The head bears a pair of inconspicuous eyes and a pair of short five-segmented antennae. The three pairs of legs are stout and well developed. The short thick tibia has a small thumb-like spine on its inner side at the apex, while the short tarsus has a curved claw (Fig. 12.2a). Hairs of the host, or his clothing, are gripped between this spine and claw.

The mouthparts of the louse are different from those of most other blood-sucking insects in that they do not constitute a projecting piercing proboscis. They consist of a flexible, sucking, almost tube-like mouth, called the haustellum, which is armed on the inner surface with minute teeth which grip the host's skin

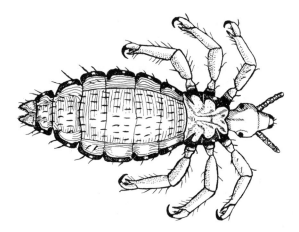

Fig. 12.1 *Pediculus humanus humanus*, the body louse. (The head louse, *P. humanus capitis*, looks virtually the same.)

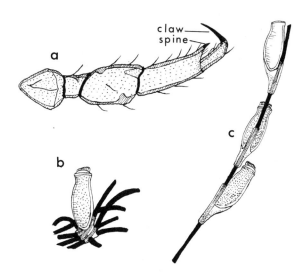

Fig. 12.2 Body and head lice. (a) Leg of *P. humanus* showing tarsal claw and tibial spine; (b) unhatched egg of body louse glued to fibres of clothing; (c) two unhatched and one hatched egg of head louse glued to hair from the head. These three eggs are for convenience shown very close together, but they are never this close in practice.

during feeding. Needle-like stylets are thrust into the skin and saliva is injected into the wound. Blood is sucked into the mouth and passes into the stomach for digestion.

The lateral margins of the abdominal segments are sclerotised and much darker than the rest of the segments. In female lice the tip of the abdomen is bifurcated and this is associated with her gripping fibres of clothing during egg laying.

Life-cycle

Both sexes take blood-meals and feeding occurs at any time during the day or night. Both the adult and immature stages live permanently on man, clinging mainly to hairs of his clothing and usually only on to body hairs during feeding. Female lice glue about 6–9 eggs per day very firmly on to the hairs of clothing, especially to those along the seams of underclothes, such as vests and pants, but also on shirts and occasionally on body hairs. The egg, commonly called a nit (though strictly this term should be applied only to the hatched egg), is oval and white, and has a distinct operculum containing numerous small perforations which give the egg the appearance of a miniscule pepper pot (Fig. 12.2b, c). The intake of air through these holes not only supplies the tissues of the developing embryo with oxygen but aids hatching in the following way. Just prior to hatching, the fully developed louse within its egg shell swallows air which distends the body against the egg shell, thus building up a back pressure causing the head of the louse to be pushed up against the operculum and forcing if off. Female lice may live for 1 month and lay 200–300 eggs.

The duration of the egg stage is normally about 6–10 days, but eggs on discarded clothing away from the warmth of the body may not hatch until 2–3 weeks. Eggs, however, cannot survive longer than 4 weeks, consequently there is little danger of infestation with body lice from clothing which has not been worn for over 1 month.

Lice have a hemimetabolous life-cycle. The louse which hatches from the egg is termed a nymph and resembles a small adult louse. It takes a blood-meal from man and passes through three nymphal instars, and after about 7–14 days becomes an adult male or female louse. The duration of the nymphal stages depends much on whether or not clothing is worn all the time. If it is discarded at night this may result in subjecting the nymphs to lower temperatures, thus slowing down their development. Each louse usually takes several blood-meals a day from its host.

The body louse is a true ectoparasite of man. Unfed lice die within about 2–5 days if kept away from man and without a blood-meal, but blood-fed individuals may survive for 5–10 days. Lice are very sensitive to changes in temperature. They quickly abandon a dead person, owing to cooling down of his body, to seek out new hosts; they also leave a person with a high temperature. They are unable to feed at temperatures above about 40°C.

A very heavily infested person may have 400–500 lice on his clothing and body. There is one record of an estimated 10 000 lice and 10 000 eggs from a single shirt! Usually, however, fewer than 100 lice are found on people, and many have considerably less than this.

Body lice are spread by close contact and are especially prevalent under conditions of overcrowding and in situations where people rarely wash or change their clothes. They are therefore commonly found on people in primitive jails, refugee camps and in trenches during wars, and also after disasters such as floods or earthquakes when people are forced to live in very overcrowded, and usually insanitary, conditions. Infestation may reach a peak in cold weather when several layers of woollen underclothes are worn and are rarely changed.

Medical importance

Pediculosis

The presence of body, head or pubic lice on a person is sometimes referred to as pediculosis. The skin of people who habitually harbour large numbers of body lice may become pigmented and tough, a condition known as vagabond's disease or sometimes as *morbus errorum*.

Because lice feed several times a day, saliva is repeatedly injected into people harbouring lice, and toxic effects may lead to weariness, irritability or a pessimistic mood, the person feels lousy. Allergies such as severe itching may be caused by repeated inoculation of saliva, and if inhaled the faeces may produce symptoms reminiscent of hay fever.

Louse-borne epidemic typhus

The rickettsiae of louse-borne typhus, *Rickettsia prowazeki*, are ingested with the blood-meal taken by both male and female lice, and also their nymphs. They invade the epithelial cells lining the stomach of the louse where they multiply enormously and cause the cells to become greatly distended. About 4 days after the blood-meal the gut cells rupture and release the rickettsiae back into the lumen of the insect's intestine. Due to these injuries to the intestinal wall, the blood-meal may seep into the haemocele of the louse, giving the body an overall reddish colour. The rickettsiae are passed out with the faeces of the louse, and man becomes infected when these are rubbed or scratched into abrasions, or come into contact with delicate mucous membranes, such as conjunctiva. Infection can also be caused by inhalation of the very fine powdered dry faeces. Alternatively, if a louse is crushed, such as by persistent scratching because of the irritation caused by its bites, the rickettsiae in the gut are released and may cause infection through abrasions, etc. The rickettsiae may remain alive and infective in dried lice faeces for 90 days.

Man, therefore, becomes infected with typhus either by the faeces of the louse or by crushing it, not by its bite. An unusual feature of louse-borne epidemic typhus is that it is a disease of the louse as well as of man. The rupturing of the epithelial cells of the intestine, caused by the multiplication of the rickettsiae, frequently kills the louse after about 8–12 days. This may explain why people suffering from typhus are sometimes found with no, or remarkably few, lice on their bodies or clothing.

Man is usually considered to be the reservoir of the disease. Asymptomatic carriers remain infective to body lice for many years. Recrudescences as Brill–Zinsser's disease, many years after the primary attack, may occur in a person and lead to the spread of epidemic typhus.

Trench fever

This is a relatively uncommon and non-fatal disease which was first noticed during World War I (1914–18) amongst soldiers in the trenches, and then reappeared again in eastern Europe during World War II (1939–45).

It is caused by *Rochalimaea quintana* which is ingested by the louse during feeding on man. The pathogens are attached to the walls of the gut cells where they multiply; they do not penetrate the cells as do typhus rickettsiae and consequently they are not injurious to the louse. After 5–10 days the faeces are infected. Like typhus, the disease is conveyed to man either by crushing the louse, or by its faeces coming into contact with skin abrasions or mucous membranes. The pathogens persist for a long time, possibly a year in dried louse faeces, and it is suspected that infection may commonly arise from inhalation of the dust-like faeces. The disease may be contracted by those who have no lice but are handling louse-infected clothing contaminated with faeces.

Louse-borne epidemic relapsing fever

The causative agent *Borrelia recurrentis* is ingested with the louse's blood-meal from a person suffering from epidemic relapsing fever. Within about 24 hours all spirochaetes have disappeared from the lumen of the gut. Many have been destroyed, but the survivors have succeeded in passing through the stomach wall to the haemocele, where they multiply greatly, reaching enormous numbers by the 10th–12th days. The only way in which man can be infected with louse-borne relapsing fever is by the louse being crushed and the released spirochaetes entering the body through abrasions or mucous membranes. The habit of some people of crushing lice between the fingernails, or the even less desirable habit of killing them by cracking them with the teeth, is clearly dangerous if the lice are infected with relapsing fever, or rickettsiae.

The method of transmission of epidemic relapsing fever must make it very rare for more than one person to be infected by any one infected louse. Hence epidemics of louse-borne relapsing fever will rarely occur unless there are large louse populations.

Control

The most obvious way to eradicate body lice from a person is by changing and washing the clothing in water hotter than 60°C, preferably followed by ironing. In epidemic situations, however, such measures may be impractical and immediate reinfestation may occur, hence insecticides are usually used for louse control.

Ten per cent DDT dust mixed with an inert carrier (talc) can be blown, at about the rate of 30 g per person, between the body and underclothes. If DDT-resistant lice are present then 1 per cent HCH powder can be used. If the lice are also resistant to this insecticide 1 per cent malathion dust should be tried. DDT resistance has developed in many countries and lice resistant to HCH are also quite common; malathion-resistant lice have also been reported. If lice are resistant to all these compounds alternative insecticidal dusts are 2 per cent temephos (Abate), 5 per cent carbaryl (Sevin), 1 per cent propoxur (Baygon) or 0·2 per cent pyrethrum. Since insecticidal dusts come into close and prolonged contact with people, it is essential that they have very low mammalian toxicities.

THE HEAD LOUSE
(*PEDICULUS HUMANUS CAPITIS*)

External morphology

There are only very minor morphological differences separating body and head lice. In practice, these differences are not very important because lice found on clothing or on the body are invariably body lice, while those on the head are nearly always head lice. In this book these two lice are regarded as subspecies, because under laboratory conditions they can interbreed. However, they are often regarded as distinct species.

Life-cycle

The life-cycle is very similar to that of the body louse except the eggs (nits) are not laid on clothes, but are cemented to the base of hairs of the head (see Fig. 12.2c), especially behind and above the ears, and the back of the neck. The distance between the scalp and the furthest egg glued to a hair provides an approximate estimate of the duration of infestation. Only very occasionally are eggs laid on hairs elsewhere on the body. Most individuals harbour only 10–20 head lice, but in very severe infestations the hair may become matted with a mixture of nits, nymphs, adults and exudates from pustules resulting from bites of the lice. In such cases bacterial and fungal infections may become established and an unpleasant crust formed on parts of the head, underneath which are masses of head lice. Empty, hatched eggs remain firmly cemented to the hairs of the head. A female lays about 6–8 eggs per day, amounting to about 150–300 eggs during her life-span, which is a little over 1 month. Eggs hatch within 7–10 days and the duration of the nymphal stages is about 7–9 days.

As with body lice, dissemination of head lice is only by close contact, such as children playing together and with their heads frequently touching, or when people are crowded together such as in prisons or refugee camps. Use of other people's hats, scarves, combs, hair brushes, etc. has not been proved to spread head lice. The occasional head louse found on such articles or on the backs of chairs are moribund individuals that will not be able to survive and infect someone else. Head lice are often rarer in men than in children or women of all ages. There is no correlation between hair length and infestation rates.

Medical importance

There is no evidence that head lice are natural vectors of the diseases transmitted by body lice—typhus epidemics are always associated with body lice. However, under experimental conditions head lice can transmit both rickettsiae and spirochaetes. Head lice can transmit impetigo; the bacteria being ingested with the blood-meal and passing out unharmed with the faeces.

Control

Regular washing with soap and warm water may reduce the numbers of nymphs and adults on the hair, but will have no effect on the eggs which are firmly glued to the bases of the hairs. Lice and nits can be removed by a steel or plastic comb, which has very closely-set fine teeth. Alternatively, the head can be shaved. Regular combing with an ordinary comb, although not removing the eggs, may reduce the number of nymphs and adults.

Insecticidal formulations for louse control include dusts, emulsions and lotions. The choice of formulation and insecticide depends on the availability of proprietary brands, preference of patients, degree of residual action required and costs. Although dusts (e.g. 10 per cent DDT and 1 per cent malathion) are efficient, they are not acceptable to most people because they give the head a greyish appearance and reveal that the person has lice. Preparations such as shampoos which are applied and then washed off after a few minutes are not usually very effective and are not recommended.

Emulsions of 2–5 per cent DDT or 0·1 per cent HCH can be used, but if head lice are resistant to these compounds then emulsions containing 1 per cent permethrin, 0·3–0·4 per cent bio-allethrin, 2 per cent temephos, 0·5 per cent malathion, propoxur (Baygon) or carbaryl (Sevin) can be applied. These insecticidal preparations should be left on the head for 12–24 hours, after which the hair can be washed.

A second washing with an insecticidal preparation after an interval of 7–10 days is required with formulations of DDT or HCH as they have no, or little, effect on the eggs. If, however, malathion or carbaryl is used, only a single treatment is required because this kills eggs as well as nymphs and adults. None of the compounds will remove eggs cemented to the hairs, but these can be removed with a louse comb.

THE PUBIC LOUSE (*PTHIRUS PUBIS*)

External morphology

The pubic louse is generally smaller (1–2 mm) than *Pediculus* and is easily distinguished from it. In the pubic louse there is less

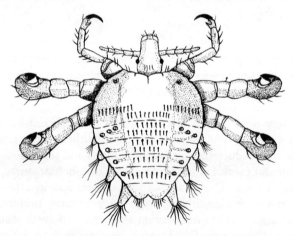

Fig. 12.3 *Pthirus pubis*, the pubic louse, showing large tarsal claws of mid and hind legs.

differentiation between the thorax and abdomen, together they are almost round so that the body is nearly as broad as long. Whereas all three pairs of legs are more or less equal in size in the body and head lice, in the pubic louse the front pair, although as long as the other two pairs, is much more slender and has smaller claws. In marked contrast, the middle and hind legs have massive claws (Fig. 12.3). The presence of a broad squat body, very large claws on the middle and hind legs, together with the characteristically more sluggish movements, has resulted in the pubic louse being aptly called the crab louse.

Life-cycle

The life-cycle is very similar to that of *Pediculus*. Eggs take about 6–8 days to hatch and the nymphal stages last about 10–17 days. Females lay a total of about 150–200 eggs which are slightly smaller than those of the body and head louse, and are cemented to the coarse hairs of the genital and perianal regions of the body. Pubic lice may be found on other areas of the body having coarse and not very dense covering of hair, for example the beard, moustache, eyelashes, underneath the arms and occasionally on the chest. They are very rarely found on the head. Pubic lice are considerably less active than *Pediculus*. The life-cycle, from egg laying to formation of the adult, is about 17–25 days.

Infestation with crab lice is usually through sexual intercourse, and characteristically the French call them 'papillons d'amour'. However, it is wrong to suspect that this is the only method. Young children sleeping with parents can catch crab lice, and infestations can arise from discarded clothing, infested bedding, or even *rarely* from lavatory seats. Adults can survive only 2 days away from their hosts.

Medical importance

Although under laboratory conditions pubic lice can transmit louse-borne typhus, there is little evidence that under natural conditions they spread any disease, although there was a suggestion that they have been responsible for typhus outbreaks in China. In some individuals, however, severe allergic reactions develop to their bites due to the injection of saliva and the deposition around the feeding sites of faeces. Small characteristic blue spots (*maculae cerulae*) may appear on the infested parts of the body. Infestations of pubic lice are sometimes known as *pediculosis pubis*.

Control

Originally control involved shaving pubic hairs from the body, but this method has been replaced by the applications of insecticidal emulsions and lotions as used for head lice control. In addition, 10 per cent DDT, 2 per cent HCH or 0·5 per cent malathion powders can be used, but powders are usually less effective than emulsions or lotions. If DDT or HCH has been used then a second treatment should be given 7–10 days later as organochlorine insecticides do not kill the eggs, and in some infestations a third treatment may be required. Formulations containing malathion or carbaryl (Sevin) are usually better, and a single efficient application should kill eggs as well as nymphs and adults.

It may be advisable to treat all hairy areas of the body below the neck. Insecticidal shampoos are ineffective for controlling pubic lice.

Some insecticides may cause irritation and dermatitis due to the sensitivity of the genital regions, in such cases shaving may remain a relatively simple and effective remedy.

Chapter 13
Bedbugs

There are two common species of bedbugs, both of which feed on man; *Cimex lectularius*, which has a widespread distribution, and *C. hemipterus*, commonly called the tropical bedbug, which is essentially a species of the Old and New World tropics, but which also occurs in temperate regions. It is not always easy to separate these two bedbugs, but in *C. lectularius* the prothorax is generally $2\frac{1}{2}$ times as wide as long, whereas in *C. hemipterus* it is only about twice as wide as long. Also, in *C. hemipterus* the abdomen is not as roundish as in *C. lectularius*.

Bedbugs are not considered important vectors, but in addition to constituting a biting nuisance, they may aid the transmission of hepatitis B virus. In India bedbugs have been reported as causing iron deficiency in infants.

External morphology

The adults are oval, wingless insects which are flattened dorso-ventrally (Fig. 13.1). They are about 4–7 mm long and when unfed a pale yellow or brown colour, but after a full blood-meal they become a characteristically darker 'mahogany' brown. The head is short and broad and has a pair of prominent compound eyes, in front of which are a pair of four-segmented antennae. The proboscis is slender, and is normally held closely appressed along the ventral surface of the head and prothorax, but when the bug takes a blood-meal it is swung forward and downwards (Fig. 13.2a). The prothorax is much larger than the meso- and meta-thorax and has distinct wing-like expansions. The rudimentary and non-functional wings, termed the hemielytra, appear as two more or less oval pads overlying the meso- and metathorax. The three pairs of legs are slender but well developed.

The abdomen is divided into eight visible segments. In adult males the tip of the abdomen is slightly more pointed than in the

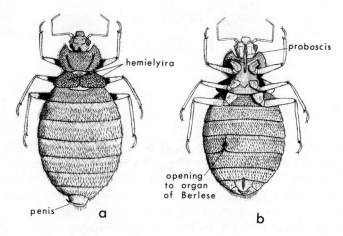

Fig. 13.1 The bedbug, *Cimex hemipterus*. (a) Dorsal view of adult male; (b) ventral view of adult female.

females and careful examination shows that there is a small well-developed and curved penis (see Fig. 13.1a). When viewed ventrally a small incision is seen on the left side of the fourth abdominal segment of females (see Fig. 13.1b). This opens into a special pouch called the mesospermalege or the organ of Berlese or Ribaga, which serves to collect and store sperm. Since both male and female bugs bite man it may not, however, be very important to distinguish the sexes.

Life-cycle

Both sexes take blood-meals and are equally important as pests. Feeding usually occurs on sleeping persons during the night, especially just before dawn, but if the bedbugs are starving, they will feed during the day in dark rooms, or sometimes in light ones. Bedbugs, unlike fleas and lice, do not stay long on man but visit him only to take blood-meals. During the day both adults and nymphs are inactive and hide away in a variety of dark and dry places, such as cracks and crevices in furniture, walls, ceilings or floorboards, underneath seams of wallpaper and between mattresses and beds. Bedbugs are gregarious and are frequently found in large numbers.

Females lay about 6–10 eggs a week which are deposited in the same places where the bugs hide, such as in cracks and crevices of buildings and furniture. The eggs are about 1 mm long, pearly or yellowish-white, covered with a very fine and delicate mosaic pattern, and characteristically slightly curved anteriorly (Fig. 13.2b). Some 500 or more eggs can sometimes be found more or less together, cemented on rough surfaces such as walls, or deposited in cracks. Females live several weeks to many months, and during this time may lay 50 to several hundred eggs.

The eggs usually hatch after about 8-11 days, but within less than a week if temperatures are about 27°C; if, however, temperatures in houses are low, hatching may be delayed for several weeks. At low temperatures eggs can survive for up to 3 months, but hatching will not occur below about 13°C. During hatching the small operculum is pushed up from the anterior end of the egg, but often remains partially attached. Empty egg shells usually remain cemented in place after hatching. The newly hatched bedbug (nymph) is very pale yellow and resembles an adult, but is much smaller (Fig. 13.2c). The life-cycle is hemimetabolous and there are five nymphal instars, each of which takes one or more blood-meals. The nymphal period commonly lasts 5-8 weeks, but may be greatly extended in cool conditions or if regular blood-feeding is prevented by lack of hosts. In the absence of man, bedbugs will feed on a variety of mammals, including rabbits, rats, mice and bats, and even on poultry and other birds. Adult bedbugs can, at least in the laboratory, live up

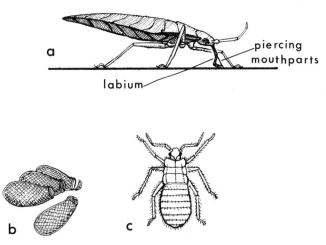

Fig. 13.2 Bedbugs. (a) Diagram of adult with proboscis swung forward for feeding; (b) one hatched and three unhatched eggs; (c) 1st-instar nymph.

to 4 years, and can withstand long periods of starvation—up to 550 days. Survival, however, is very much dependent on temperature and humidity.

The method of mating in bedbugs is unique amongst insects. The penis is not introduced into the genital opening, but penetrates the integument and enters the organ of Berlese (organ of Ribaga or mesospermalege) situated on the ventral surface of the female. This organ serves as a copulatory pouch into which spermatozoa are introduced. After 1 or 2 hours spermatozoa leave this 'pouch' and pass into the haemocele of the female, and then migrate to the bases of the oviducts and ascend to the ovaries where fertilisation occurs.

Bedbugs in houses can be detected by the presence of live bugs, the cast-off skins of the nymphs, and hatched and unhatched eggs, all of which may be found in cracks and crevices. In addition, small dark brown or black marks may be visible on bed sheets, walls and wallpaper, these are the bedbug's excreta and consist mainly of excess blood ingested during feeding. Houses with heavy infestations of bedbugs may have a characteristic sweet and rather sickly smell, but in practice this may not be apparent because the weak odour is masked by stronger insanitary smells. At night male and female adults, and nymphs, crawl from their daytime resting places to feed on sleeping people, after which they return to their resting sites to digest their blood-meals. Bedbugs can move quite rapidly when disturbed.

Bedbugs have limited powers of dispersal because they do not have wings. Occasionally they may crawl from one building to another, but they usually spread to new houses by being introduced with furniture and bedding, or more rarely with clothing and hand baggage. Buying secondhand furniture can result in the introduction of bedbugs into houses.

Medical importance

In the past bedbugs have not been considered to transmit disease to man, but in Africa hepatitis B virus has been recorded from bedbugs. It seems possible that the virus could be spread through contaminated faeces being scratched into abrasions, or even by inhalation of faecal dusts.

In some areas, especially those with dilapidated buildings and low standards of hygiene, bedbug infestations can cause considerable distress. Reaction to their bites is variable. Some people show little or no reaction while others may suffer severe reactions and sleepless nights. In India repeated feedings of large numbers of bedbugs has been reported as responsible for iron deficiency in infants.

Control

Floors and walls of infested houses together with as much furniture as possible should be sprayed with 5 per cent DDT emulsion. If, however, bedbugs are resistant to DDT then 0·5 per cent HCH should be tried, and if the bugs are also resistant to this compound, other insecticides such as 1–2 per cent malathion, 0·5 per cent diazinon or 0·5 per cent dichlorvos (DDVP) can be used. The addition of 0·1–0·2 per cent pyrethrins or synthetic pyrethroids, such as bioresmethrin, to sprays is useful because it helps flush out bedbugs from their hiding places and thus increases their contact with the insecticide.

Bedding and mattresses can be lightly sprayed with insecticides (not diazinon), but should be aired afterwards to allow them to dry out completely before being re-used. Insecticidal dusts can also be applied to mattresses and bedding. Infants' bedding should not be treated with insecticides. Commercially available insecticide smoke generators (usually containing HCH or DDT) can be useful for fumigating infested premises.

Chapter 14
Triatomine Bugs

The blood-sucking species of reduviid bugs belong to the subfamily Triatominae which comprises 14 genera and some 111 species. Principal species of medical importance are *Rhodnius prolixus*, *Panstrongylus megistus* and species of *Triatoma* such as *T. infestans*, and *T. dimidiata*, all of which spread Chagas' disease (*Trypanosoma cruzi*) in Central and South America. They also transmit *Trypanosoma rangeli*, an apparently non-pathogenic organism.

Most Triatominae occur in the Americas, ranging from the southern States of the USA to Argentina, but a few species are found in the Old World tropics. All medically important species are confined to the southern USA, Central and South America. They are commonly called cone-nose bugs, assassin bugs or kissing bugs.

External morphology

These bugs vary in size from about 0·5–4·5 cm, but most are 2–3 cm long. They are easily recognised by their long snout-like head which bears a pair of prominent dark-coloured eyes, in front of which are a pair of laterally situated, long and thin four-segmented antennae (Fig. 14.1). The proboscis, sometimes called the rostrum, is relatively thin and straight and, as in bedbugs, lies closely appressed to the ventral surface of the head (Fig. 14.2a). When the Triatominae take a blood-meal the proboscis is swung forward and downwards (Fig. 14.2b). Bugs in other subfamilies of the Reduviidae are predacious on small insects and the proboscis is usually thicker and more robust than in the Triatominae, and is distinctly curved. Another difference is that the antennae arise from the dorsal surface of the head and not from its sides as in the blood-sucking Triatominae.

The dorsal part of the first segment of the thorax of the Triatominae consists of a very conspicuous triangular pronotum. The

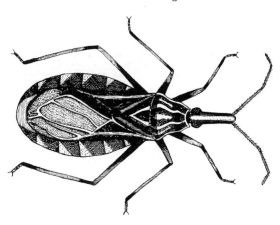

Fig. 14.1 Adult *Rhodnius*, as example of a triatomine bug.

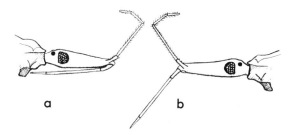

Fig. 14.2 Lateral view of head of *Rhodnius* showing proboscis. (a) Proboscis closely appressed to ventral side of head; (b) proboscis swung forward in feeding position.

meso- and metathorax are completely hidden dorsally by the folded forewings which are called hemielytra. The basal part of each hemielytron is thickened and relatively hard, whereas the more distal part is membranous (Fig. 14.3). The hindwings are entirely membranous but when the bug is not flying they remain hidden underneath the hemielytra. The thorax has three pairs of relatively long and slender legs which end in paired small claws.

The abdomen is more or less oval in shape but is mostly covered by the wings, except for the lateral margins which are bent upwards slightly and are visible dorsally.

Triatominae are frequently a rather dull brown-black colour, but some species are more colourful having contrasting yellow or

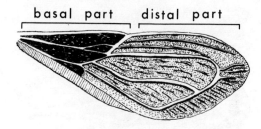

Fig. 14.3 Forewing, or hemielytron, of a triatomine bug showing thickened basal part, and membraneous distal part.

red markings, usually present as bands on the pronotum, basal part of the forewings or margins of the abdomen.

Life-cycle

Eggs are deposited in or near the habitation of their hosts, such as in cracks and crevices in walls, floors, ceilings and furniture of houses, especially old dilapidated mud-walled and thatched-roofed houses in rural areas, or slums at the edge of towns. Adults also lay their eggs in rodent burrows and a variety of shelters used by mammalian hosts upon which the bugs feed. Some species feed on birds and deposit their eggs in birds' nests and on leaves of trees. Eggs are about 1·5–2·5 mm long, pink, yellowish or white in colour depending on the species, and have a smooth shell. They are oval in shape but have a slight constriction before the operculum (Fig. 14.4). Some species lay eggs in small batches which may be glued to the substrate, others lay them more or less singly, either free or cemented to the substrate. The total number of eggs laid by females varies between about 50–1000, usually 200–300, depending on the species, their longevity and the number of blood-meals they take. The life-cycle is hemimetabolous.

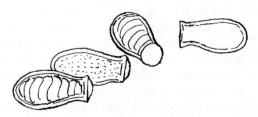

Fig. 14.4 Hatched and unhatched triatomine eggs.

Small pale nymphs, which resemble adults but lack wings, may hatch from the eggs after only 10–15 days, but the incubation period may extend to 30, or even 60, days. These newly emerged nymphs usually remain hidden in cracks and crevices for a few days before they seek out blood-meals. There are five nymphal instars, each instar requires at least one complete blood-meal before it changes into a succeeding one. Rudimentary wing pads begin to be clearly visible in the fourth and fifth nymphal stages, but only adults have fully developed functional wings. Young nymphs can ingest as much as twelve times their own weight of blood, and as a result their abdomens may become so greatly distended that they resemble blood-red balloons. Successive instars take relatively less blood, so that the fifth and last nymphal stage takes about three to five times its own weight of blood, and adults ingest about twice their weight of blood. Sometimes hungry nymphs and adult bugs pierce the swollen abdomens of freshly engorged nymphs and take a blood-meal from them without apparently causing any harm.

Nymphs and adults of both sexes feed at night on their hosts, and feeding is a lengthy process lasting 10–25 minutes or more. When people are covered with blankets the bugs feed on exposed parts of the body such as the nose and around the eyes and mouth, but in hot weather they will readily feed on other exposed areas of the body. Bites are usually relatively painless and do not awaken people, but some species cause considerable discomfort and there may be prolonged after-effects. Many Triatominae defecate during feeding and this behaviour is very important in the transmission of Chagas' disease.

Because of the relatively long time required, even under optimum laboratory conditions, to digest their large blood-meals, the life-cycle from egg to adult takes at least 3–3½ months but more usually 6–10 months. Under natural conditions it often takes about 1 year, but sometimes the life-cycle is 2 years. In the absence of hosts, older nymphs and adults can survive 4–6 months of starvation.

Species of bugs in the subfamily Triatominae inhabit both forests and drier areas of the Americas. Many species feed on a variety of wild animals, such as armadillos, opossums, rats, mice, marsupials, ground squirrels, skunks, iguanas, bats, and also birds. Adults and nymphs are usually found in the burrows or nests of these animals. In addition to these sylvatic species,

certain bugs have become highly domesticated and feed on animals
such as donkeys, cattle, goats, horses, pigs, cats, dogs and especially chickens, which in some areas appear to be particularly
important hosts, and of course man. These domestic species often
live in man-made shelters including houses, especially primitive
ones made of wood, mud and thatch. Some species are partially
sylvatic and domestic in their feeding and resting habits. Sylvatic
species sometimes readily move into houses from the forest as it
is cut down and man occupies previously uninhabited areas.

   If hosts vacate their shelters or homes, hungry nymphs eventually crawl out from their hiding places to seek new hosts, while
adults, which are strong fliers, fly out to find new hosts and
shelters. Some species are attracted into houses by lights.

Medical importance

Chagas' disease

Triatominae are of medical importance because they are vectors
of *Trypanosoma cruzi*, the causative agent of Chagas' disease,
sometimes referred to as American trypanosomiasis. Parasites
ingested with a blood-meal from a man undergo their entire development within the gut of the bug. After 9–17 days, sometimes
longer, infective metacyclic trypomastigotes (metatrypanosomes)
of *T. cruzi* are present in the lumen of the hind gut. Bugs may
also become infected by feeding on recently engorged nymphs.
Blood-feeding commonly lasts 10–25 minutes or longer, and during this time, or soon afterwards, many species of bugs excrete
liquid or semi-liquid faeces which may be contaminated with the
metacyclic forms of *T. cruzi* derived from a previous blood-meal.
Man becomes infected when the excreta is scratched either into
abrasions in the skin or in the site of the bug's bite, or when it
gets rubbed into the eyes or other mucous membranes. If the
bug's bite produces local irritation causing the person to scratch,
this facilitates infection. Transmission is not by the bite of the
insect, solely through its faeces.

   It appears that all Triatominae of the Western hemisphere can
transmit Chagas' disease, and about 66 species have already been
recorded naturally infected; but some strains of *T. cruzi* are unable
to develop in the gut of some species. In practice, however, only

those species (about 36) that have adapted to living in close association with man, and therefore regularly feed on him, are important vectors. The efficiency of a vector will also depend on the speed of feeding and whether or not the bug defecates on a person during feeding.

Chagas' disease is a zoonosis. *T. cruzi* is essentially a parasite of wild animals, such as opossums (especially *Didelphis* spp.), armadillos, many species of wild and urban rats and mice, squirrels, carnivores, monkeys and possibly bats, all of which may serve as reservoirs of infection for man. The bug itself is also a reservoir of infection, and in some areas man is considered to be the principal one. Apart from acquiring infections with *T. cruzi* through faeces, some animals become infected by eating the bugs, or by eating infected animals, such as carnivores eating rodents infected with *T. cruzi*. Man can also become infected by eating infected meat (e.g. inadequately cooked opossums) or food contaminated with excrement of infected mammals.

The infection rates of Triatominae are often exceptionally high. For example, it is not uncommon to find infection rates of about 25 or even 40 per cent or more. Even higher infection rates (78 per cent) have been found in *Triatoma protracta* in California, but because this species very rarely bites man it is not considered a vector to humans.

Trypanosoma rangeli

Another trypanosome, *Trypanosoma rangeli*, which is apparently non-pathogenic in man, is also transmitted by the Triatominae including *T. infestans* and *T. dimidiata*, but the most important vector is *Rhodnius prolixus*. In the insect vector the trypanosomes undergo dual development, some of the metacyclic infective forms migrate to the hind gut but others penetrate the gut wall, pass across into the haemocele and then migrate to the salivary glands. Man is infected by both the bug's faeces and bite, but the latter seems to be the most important method of transmission, and some have questioned whether infection ever arises from the bug's faeces.

A few arboviruses have been recovered from the Triatominae, but they have not been incriminated as important vectors of any diseases other than Chagas' disease.

Control

The usual control methods consist of applying residual insecticides to the interior surfaces of walls and roofs of houses. The most common formulation is a water-dispersable powder of 1·25 per cent HCH applied at the rate of 0·5 g/m². 2·5 per cent dieldrin at a dosage of 1 g/m² is also effective, but careless handling by spray men has resulted in cases of poisoning. HCH remains effective for only about 1 month, whereas dieldrin persists for 2–3 months. DDT has mainly proved ineffective, because of the development of resistance. Alternative insecticides which have shown promise include propoxur (Baygon) and malathion. House-spraying will only destroy bugs resting in houses, it will not kill those resting in natural outdoor shelters and, depending on the area and habits of the species of Triatominae biting man, these outdoor populations may be important in the transmission of Chagas' disease. The spraying of houses with residual insecticides in malaria control campaigns has frequently reduced populations of Triatominae and the incidence of Chagas' disease.

Replacement of mud and thatched dilapidated houses with those built of brick or cement blocks and corrugated metal roofs should significantly contribute towards the elimination of domestic bugs. However, because of the high cost of such measures, rehousing has not been carried out on a sufficiently large scale for it to produce any significant impact on transmission, except on a local basis.

Chapter 15
Cockroaches

There are almost 4000 species of cockroaches. About 50 species have become domestic pests, and the most important medically are *Blattella germanica* (the German cockroach), *Blatta orientalis* (the Oriental cockroach) and *Periplaneta americana* (the American cockroach). Cockroaches are sometimes called roaches or steam-bugs. They have a world-wide distribution.

Cockroaches almost certainly aid in the transmission and harbourage of various pathogenic viruses, bacteria, protozoa and helminths. They can be intermediate hosts of certain nematodes, and an acanthocephalid which rarely parasitises man.

External morphology

The following general description refers to the more common household pest species. They are usually chestnut brown or black in colour, about 1·5–4·5 cm long, flattened dorsoventrally and have a smooth, shiny and tough integument. Viewed from above the head appears small, and it is sometimes almost hidden by the large, rounded pronotum. A pair of long and prominent filiform antennae arise from the front of the head between the eyes (Fig. 15.1). The cockroach mouthparts are developed for chewing, gnawing and scraping, they are not composed of piercing stylets and therefore cockroaches cannot suck blood. In adults of both sexes there are two pairs of wings. In certain household species those in the female may be shorter than those of the male, and in female *Blatta orientalis* they are very small and non-functional. The forewings are rather leathery and are called tegima; they are not used in flight but serve as protective covers for the hindwings, which are membranous and can be used for flying, but when not in use are folded shut fan-like over the body. Although cockroaches possess wings they rarely fly in temperate climates. There are three pairs of legs which are well developed and covered with

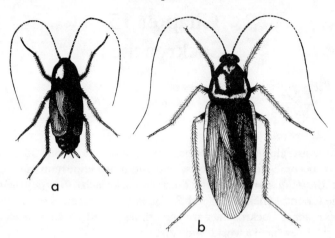

Fig. 15.1   Adult cockroaches. (a) *Blatta orientalis*; (b) *Periplaneta americana*.

prominent small spines and bristles; they terminate in a pair of
claws.

The segmented abdomen is more or less oval in shape but is
either completely or partly hidden from view, depending on the
species, by the folded overlapping wings. In both sexes a pair of
prominent segmented pilose cerci arise from the last abdominal
segment (Fig. 15.2a), but they are hidden from view in some
species by the wings.

Cockroaches are most readily distinguished from beetles (order
Coleoptera) by having the forewings placed over the abdomen in
a scissor-like manner. In beetles the forewings (elytra) are not
crossed over but meet dorsally to form a distinct line down the
centre of the abdomen. In addition, the elytra of beetles are
generally stouter than the tegima of cockroaches.

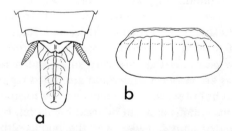

Fig. 15.2   (a) Ootheca protruding from the abdomen of *Blattella germanica*;
(b) typical cockroach ootheca.

gationCockroaches211

Life-cycle

Cockroaches like warmth and during the day they hide away behind radiators and hot-water pipes, and in warm countries where these may be absent, in almost any dark place, such as cesspits, septic tanks, sewers, rubbish dumps, refuse tips, dustbins, cupboards, drawers, underneath chairs, tables, sinks, baths and beds, behind refrigerators, cooking stoves, dishes in kitchens—in fact in almost any dark place. They are usually common in kitchens especially if remains of food are left out overnight. They abound in restaurants, hotels, bakeries, breweries, laundries and on ships. They are also found throughout the world in hospitals. Cockroaches are nocturnal in habit and are rarely seen during the day unless they are disturbed from their hiding places. They become very active at night, crawling over floors, tables and other furniture to seek food. They move very quickly and can be both seen and heard scuttling along when lights are suddenly switched on.

They are omnivorous and voracious feeders, any type of man's food is eaten. They also consume paper, clothes, particularly starched ones, books, hair, shoes, wallpaper, dried blood, sputum, excreta, dead insects, and almost any animal or vegetable matter. They have been recorded gnawing at the finger and toe-nails of sleeping or comatose people, and on vagabonds even infesting the hair. They habitually disgorge partially digested food and deposit their excreta on almost anything, including food. Cockroaches may live for 5–10 weeks without water and for many months without food, but in practice this is not an important limiting factor because they very rarely occur in areas where food of some kind is not available. Young nymphs, however, may die within about 7–10 days in the absence of food.

Eggs are laid encased in a brown bean-shaped case or capsule called an ootheca (Fig. 15.2b) which contains 14–48 eggs. Cockroaches are often seen running around with an ootheca partly protruding from the tip of the abdomen. The oothecae are deposited in cracks and crevices in dark and secluded places. In some species they are cemented to surfaces such as the undersides of tables, chairs and beds.

Adult cockroaches live for many months to a year or more, and during this time the female will lay about 4–90 oothecae, the number varying considerably according to species. Cockroaches have a hemimetabolous life-cycle. Nymphs hatch from the eggs after about 1–3 months, the time depending on both temperature and species. Young nymphs are very pale and delicate versions of the adults, while the older ones are progressively darker and resemble the adults more. The nymphs are wingless, the wings gradually develop with ensuing nymphal instars, but only adults may have fully developed wings. There are usually six nymphal instars, but in *Periplaneta americana* there may be as many as 13 nymphal instars. The duration of the nymphal stage varies according to temperature, abundance of food and species. For example, the nymphal stage may occupy only about 2–3 months in *Blattella germanica*, 12–15 months in *Blatta orientalis*, and up to 10–23 months in *Periplaneta americana*. Under less ideal conditions the nymphal period of *B. germanica* extends to 6 months, and up to about 3 years in *P. americana*.

Cockroaches spread very rapidly from infested houses to adjoining ones. They often gain entry by climbing up water pipes and waste pipes. They are also spread as oothecae, nymphs and adults in furniture and other belongings.

Medical importance

The presence of cockroaches in houses and hotels, etc. has for a long time been regarded as highly undesirable because of their dirty habits of feeding indiscriminately on both excreta and foods, and their practice of excreting and regurgitating their partially digested meals over food. Because of these insanitary habits they have been suspected as aiding the transmission of various illnesses. For example, they are known to carry pathogenic viruses such as poliomyelitis, protozoa such as *Entamoeba histolytica*, *Trichomonas hominis*, *Giardia intestinalis* and *Balantidium coli*, and bacteria such as *Escherichia coli*, *Staphylococcus aureus*, *Klebsiella pneumoniae*, *Shigella dysentariae* and *Salmonella* species, including *S. typhi* and *S. typhimurium*. They are also known to be intermediate hosts of the acanthocephalid, *Moniliformis moniliformis*, which is common in rodents and can also infect cats and dogs, and very rarely man. Nematodes such as *Gonglyonema pulchrum*, a common parasite of herbivores and occasionally man, and *Enterobius vermicularis* which is an extremely common worm in man can also be carried by cockroaches. They have also been found naturally infected with *Toxoplasma gondi* and suspected of transmitting this parasite to cats, and possibly to man, by feeding on cats' faeces.

There is little doubt that cockroaches contribute to the spread of a number of diseases, mainly intestinal, and they may sometimes be more important as mechanical vectors than houseflies. However, it is nevertheless difficult to assess their real importance as vectors, because many of the pathogens which cockroaches carry can be transmitted by many other different ways.

Some people are allergic to cockroaches. It appears that sensitised people can react to cockroach allergens by eating cockroach-contaminated food, or by inhaling their dried faecal pellets.

Control

Ensuring that neither food nor dirty kitchen utensils are left out overnight will help reduce the number of cockroaches, but if they are present in adjoining or nearby houses, good hygiene in itself will not prevent cockroaches from entering houses.

Insecticidal spraying or dusting of selected sites such as cupboards, wardrobes, kitchen furniture and fixtures, underneath sinks, stoves, refrigerators, and nearby dustbins, is recommended. Unfortunately, *Blattella germanica* is almost universally resistant to most organochlorines and therefore for general purposes it is best to use 0·5 per cent sprays or 1-2 per cent dusts of organophosphate insecticides, such as fenthion (Baytex), malathion, diazinon, chlorpyrifos (Dursban) or dichlorvos (DDVP), or carbamates such as propoxur (Baygon) or carbaryl (Sevin). Sprays based on kerosene (paraffin) may leave unsightly stains on walls, and these are of course dangerous near naked flames or cookers. The residual efficiency of sprays greatly depends on the surfaces on which they are applied, for example on most painted and shiny surfaces residual activity often lasts only about 1-4 weeks. The residual action of insecticidal dusts is less affected by the nature of the surface, but dusting is unsightly and therefore objected to by many householders. The addition of pyrethrum or synthetic pyrethroids to insecticidal sprays or aerosols is useful because it irritates cockroaches and flushes them out from their hiding places. Synthetic pyrethroids such as bioresmethrin or deltamethrin applied as a spray, or more effectively as an aerosol, can produce spectacular results in flushing out and killing cockroaches.

The newer pyrethroids, such as permethrin, have the advantage of also being residual insecticides, but as yet they have been little used in cockroach control. Pyrethrum formulations, however, especially dusts, may cause allergic reactions in some people.

The best control is obtained by the applications of both sprays and dusts of the same, or different, insecticides. Boric acid powder (borax) still remains a very safe and useful chemical, acting both as a contact insecticide and a stomach poison. Sodium fluoride, although highly poisonous, is sometimes still used in poison baits for cockroach control.

Most organophosphate and carbamate insecticides can be added (1 per cent) to baits which are eaten by cockroaches and so cause their death. The addition of glycerol to poison baits provides an additional feeding stimulus.

Chapter 16
Soft Ticks

Soft ticks (Argasidae) have a more or less world-wide distribution. There are some 150 species belonging to five genera, but the medically important soft ticks belong to the genus *Ornithodoros*. The most important vector species belongs to the *Ornithodoros moubata* complex. They are vectors of tick-borne (endemic) relapsing fever caused by *Borrelia duttoni*.

External morphology

Adults are flattened dorsoventrally and oval in outline, but the shape varies according to the species. The integument is tough and leathery, wrinkled and usually has fine tubercles or granulations. There is no scutum or dorsal shield as is found in ixodid (hard) ticks. The mouthparts termed the capitulum, or 'false head', are situated ventrally (Fig. 16.1b) and thus not visible dorsally. This character serves to separate adult and nymphal soft ticks from hard ticks (Ixodidae), which have the capitulum projecting forward and clearly visible dorsally. The four-segmented palps are leg-like and the chelicerae have smooth, not denticulate,

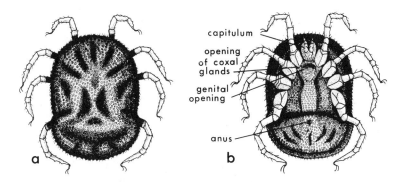

Fig. 16.1 Adults of *Ornithodoros moubata*, (a) dorsal view; (b) ventral view.

215

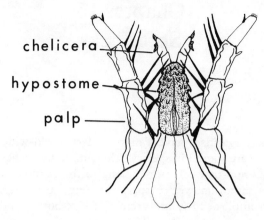

Fig. 16.2 Capitulum of an adult *Ornithodoros* species showing leg-like palps and non-denticulate cheliceral sheaths.

sheaths (Fig. 16.2). The powerful cutting chelicerae have strong teeth at their tips and together with the hypostome penetrate the host during feeding.

The four pairs of well-developed legs terminate in a pair of claws. The coxal organs (glands) open between the bases of the coxae of the first and second pairs of legs (see Fig. 16.1b).

Males and females are very similar in external appearance, but as both sexes feed on blood and can consequently be disease vectors, it is not so important to be able to distinguish between them.

Internal anatomy

A brief account of the internal anatomy of a tick is necessary in order to understand the mechanisms of disease transmission.

During feeding, saliva, which often contains powerful anticoagulants, is secreted by a pair of large grape-like salivary glands and flows down the mouthparts. Blood from the host then passes up the mouthparts, through the narrow oesophagus and into the stomach or mid gut, which is provided with numerous branching diverticula. The ramifications of the diverticula enable the adult tick to ingest large volumes of blood (about six to eight times its own weight), resulting in great distension of the tick's body. The hind gut may be absent, or be represented by a very thin and rudimentary cord-like structure.

Argasid ticks have a pair of coxal organs, which although sometimes called coxal glands, are not actually glandular but filter off excess fluid and salts from ingested blood-meals. This fluid is passed out through a small opening located between the bases of the first two pairs of legs. When a soft tick is infected with tick-borne relapsing fever (*Borrelia duttoni*) many of the spirochaetes in the haemolymph enter the coxal organs and are then passed out through their openings.

Coxal organs are present only in soft ticks, not in hard ticks.

In females of both soft and hard ticks a peculiar structure termed Gene's organ is located in front of the mid gut, and during oviposition is extruded from a small opening above the capitulum. It secretes waxy waterproofing substances which coat the eggs during oviposition and thus enables them to withstand desiccation, immersion in water and other adverse environmental conditions.

Life-cycle

A blood-meal is essential for maturation of the ovaries and egg laying. After each blood-meal female argasid ticks lay several (often 4–6) small egg batches, each of about 15–100 spherical eggs. Occasionally fewer but larger egg batches comprising as many as 200–300 eggs are laid. Adult ticks can live for many years, so a female may lay thousands of eggs during her life-time. Eggs are deposited in or near the resting places of the adult ticks, such as in cracks and crevices in the walls, floors and furniture of houses, or in mud, dust and debris, in rodent holes or in the more exposed resting or sleeping places of wild animals and birds.

Eggs hatch usually within 1–4 weeks, but because they have been coated during oviposition with a protective waxy secretion from Gene's organ (see above) they can remain viable for many months under adverse climatic conditions.

Both argasid and ixodid ticks have a hemimetabolous life-cycle, that is eggs hatch to produce six-legged larvae which superficially resemble the adults, and which moult to produce eight-legged nymphs which resemble even more closely the adults. In argasid ticks the six-legged larva (Fig. 16.3) is usually very active and searches for a host from which to take a blood-meal. The capitulum projects from the body and is visible from above. Blood-feeding on the host lasts about 20–30 minutes after which the

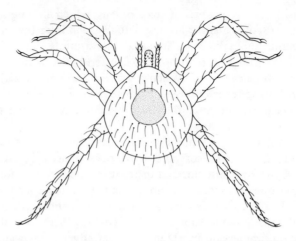

Fig. 16.3 Larva of *Argas* species, as example of typical soft tick, showing capitulum projecting in front of body.

engorged larva drops to the ground and after a few days moults to produce an eight-legged nymph. The nymph seeks out a host and feeds for about 20–30 minutes before it falls to the ground. Argasid ticks usually have four or five nymphal instars (Fig. 16.4), but up to eight in some species. Each nymphal stage requires a blood-meal before it can proceed to the next nymphal instar.

Larvae of the *Ornithodoros moubata* complex differ from most other argasid ticks in that they do not take blood-meals but remain within their egg shells after hatching, moulting to produce first-instar nymphs which crawl from the egg shells to seek their blood-meals.

The duration of the life-cycle, from egg hatching to adult, depends on the species of tick, temperature and the availability of blood-meals, but is often about 6–12 months. Adult soft ticks can live for several years, up to 15 years in the laboratory, and they can remain alive for 5 years or more after a single blood-meal. In the absence of suitable hosts argasid ticks can also survive long periods of starvation.

The distribution of the larvae, nymphs and adults of argasid ticks is usually patchy and restricted to the homes, nests and resting places of their hosts, but in these places there can be quite large populations of ticks. Species which commonly feed on man, such as some members of the *Ornithodoros moubata* complex in

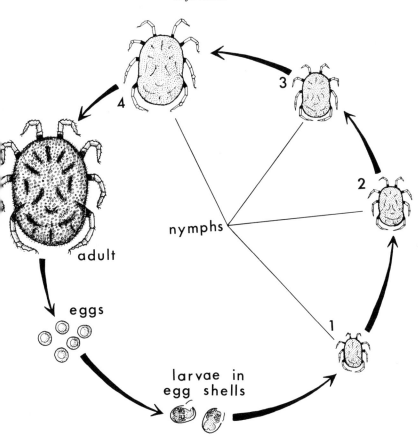

Fig. 16.4 Diagrammatic representation of the life-cycle of *Ornithodoros moubata* showing larvae retained in egg shells, and four nymphal stages.

Africa, are found around human settlements especially in village huts. However, in many parts of Africa these ticks are becoming uncommon. This may be due to changes in life-style, in particular to the increased numbers of people sleeping on beds raised from the floor, which makes it more difficult for the ticks to feed on man.

Because the larvae and all nymphal instars and adults take blood, but nevertheless remain attached for only relatively short periods, many hosts, comprising both different species and individuals, are fed upon during their life-cycle. Argasid ticks are consequently referred to as 'many-host' or 'multi-host' ticks.

Medical importance

Tick-borne relapsing fever

Soft ticks can inflict painful bites but they do not cause tick paralysis in man, as do some hard ticks (see p. 230). Tick-borne relapsing fever is the only important disease transmitted to man by soft ticks. This infection occurs throughout most of the tropics, subtropics and in many areas of the temperate regions such as North America and Europe, but it is absent from Australia and New Zealand.

The causative agent is *Borrelia duttoni*. Some authorities recognise this as a complex of different antigenic forms and have named different spirochaete species as causing relapsing fever in different parts of the world. In the present book, however, all populations and forms of the disease are assigned to a single species *Borrelia duttoni*.

Spirochaetes ingested with a blood-meal multiply in the gut and congregate along the wall of the tick's mid gut and then pass across into the haemocele where they can be found after 24 hours. In the haemocele the spirochaetes multiply enormously and invade nearly all tissues and organs of the tick's body. Within 3 days they begin to arrive in the salivary glands, the coxal organs and ovaries. In the *O. moubata* complex the salivary glands in the nymphs appear to be more heavily infected than do those of the adults in which the infection tends to diminish and die out. In contrast the coxal organs of the nymphs are usually only lightly infected whereas those of the adults become heavily infected. When either the immature stages or adults of *O. moubata* complex feed on man, or some other host, saliva is injected intermittently into the bite and spirochaetes can be introduced by this route, especially by nymphal ticks. During feeding excess body fluids are filtered from the haemocele by the coxal organs and in infected ticks, especially adults, the coxal fluids contain spirochaetes ingested with a previous blood-meal. These can enter the host through the puncture of the tick's bite or through the intact skin. Man can therefore become infected with *B. duttoni* by either, or both, the bite of *O. moubata* complex and the coxal fluids.

In other *Ornithodoros* species changes in the level of spirochaete infection with age in the salivary glands and coxal organs does not necessarily follow the same pattern. Moreover, other *Ornitho-*

doros species tend to excrete excess fluids only when they have left their host, and hence transmission by these species is mainly by the bites of the ticks. In no species of *Ornithodoros* is infection spread by faeces.

The tick itself is usually regarded as the most important reservoir, especially as there is hereditary (transovarial) transmission. The ovaries of adult female ticks become infected with spirochaetes which are then passed on to the eggs so that the newly hatched larvae, and all nymphal instars and adults of both sexes, are infected. Thus, although the larvae, nymphs and adults may not have fed on a host infected with *B. duttoni* they can nevertheless be infected and transmit the disease to other hosts. This phenomenon is called transovarial transmission and can be continued for some three to four generations.

Another rather similar and associated method of transmission is transstadial transmission. This involves one of the immature stages of a tick become infected by biting a host and then passing the infection on to one or more later stages. For example, a larva might become infected by feeding on an infected host and pass the spirochaetes to the nymphs and adults, or the infection might start with a nymph and be passed to subsequent nymphal instars and the adults. In all cases transovarial transmission can follow.

Q-fever

This is a rickettsial disease caused by *Coxiella burneti*. It has a more or less world-wide distribution and is primarily an infection of rodents and other small mammals and domestic livestock. It can be readily transmitted to people who consume contaminated milk and other foods, and also by the bites of argasid, but mainly ixodid, ticks. Transovarial transmission occurs.

Viruses

Only about 27 per cent of the 70 or so viruses known to be transmitted by ticks have been isolated from soft ticks, and very few infect man. Soft ticks, in marked contrast to hard ticks, are not regarded as important medical vectors of arboviruses. (*Ornithodoros* species, however, are the main vectors of African swine fever virus amongst pigs.)

Control

Ticks can be removed by pulling them from their hosts, but this is not always easy, especially with ixodids. It is sometimes recommended that the capitulum is compressed and pushed deeper into the skin to loosen the grip of the teeth of the hypostome, and thus prevent the body being torn off whilst the capitulum remains embedded in the host's tissues. If this happens considerable irritation and secondary infections may result. The glowing end of a cigarette often stimulates a tick to withdraw its mouthparts. Alternatively, ticks can be coated with castor oil or medicinal paraffin, Vaseline or nail varnish which prevents respiration through the spiracles and causes them slowly to release their hold so that they can be removed; or they drop off some hours later. Often the best method for removing ticks is to dab them with chloroform, ether, ethyl acetate, benzene or some other anaesthetic before carefully pulling them off.

Suitable repellents such as dimethyl phthalate, dibutyl phthalate, dimethyl carbate, butyl mesityloxide oxalate (indalone), diethyltoluamide and benzyl benzoate can be used on the skin. Alternatively, clothing can be impregnated with these chemicals, or ethyl hexanediol, to help prevent tick infestations.

Houses infested with argasid ticks such as *Ornithodoros* species can be sprayed with oil solutions or emulsions of insecticides such as 5 per cent DDT, 3 per cent malathion, 5 per cent carbaryl (Sevin), 0·5 per cent naled (Dibrom), 0·5 per cent diazinon or 1 per cent propoxur (Baygon). Special care should be taken to spray floors, and cracks and crevices in walls and furniture, and any other sites where ticks may be resting. In areas where houses have been sprayed with residual insecticides for malaria campaigns there has often been a corresponding reduction in the number of *Ornithodoros* species.

Chapter 17
Hard Ticks

Hard ticks (Ixodidae) have a world-wide distribution, but they occur more frequently in temperate regions than soft ticks (Argasidae). There are about 650 species of hard ticks belonging to 13 genera. From the medical point of view the more important genera are *Ixodes*, *Dermacentor*, *Amblyomma*, *Haemaphysalis*, and *Hyalomma*. Hard ticks are vectors of typhuses such as Rocky Mountain spotted fever (*Rickettsia rickettsii*) and *Boutonneuse* fever (*R. conori*). In addition they can spread Q-fever (*Coxiella burneti*) and many arboviruses—including Russian spring-summer encephalitis, tick-borne encephalitis, Omsk haemorrhagic fever, Kyasanur Forest disease, Colorado tick fever, and Crimean-Congo haemorrhagic fever. They also transmit tularaemia (*Pasteurella tularensis*), and cause tick paralysis.

External morphology

Adult hard ticks are flattened dorsoventrally and are oval in shape, measuring from about 3-23 mm in length depending on

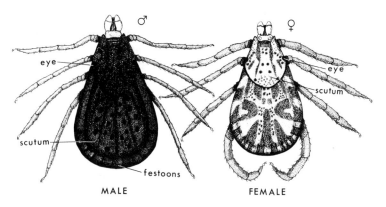

Fig. 17.1 Adults of male and female *Dermacentor* species, showing sexual differences in size of scutum. Festoons are present.

223

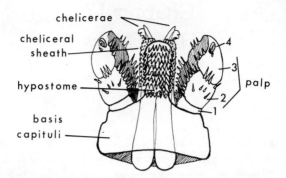

Fig. 17.2 Capitulum of an adult ixodid tick showing club-shaped palps with very minute 4th segment, and denticulate cheliceral sheaths.

species and whether they are unfed, or fully engorged with blood. The females are nearly always bigger than the males, and because they take larger blood-meals they enlarge much more than males during feeding.

The capitulum or 'false head' projects forwards beyond the body outline and is visible from above (Fig 17.1), thus distinguishing adult hard (ixodid) ticks from soft (argasid) ticks (see Fig. 16.1). There are also differences in the shape and structure of the capitulum which serves to separate the two families. For example, in hard ticks the palps are swollen and club-shaped (Fig. 17.2) rather than leg-shaped as in the soft ticks. The toothed hypostome is located between a pair of chelicerae, which, unlike those of soft ticks, have their cheliceral sheaths covered with very small denticles, giving them what is sometimes termed a 'shagreened' appearance. As in argasid ticks both the hypostome and chelicerae penetrate the host during feeding.

The posterior margin of the body in species of the genera *Dermacentor*, *Rhipicephalus* and *Haemaphysalis* has a number of rectangular indentations called 'festoons'. However, in fully engorged females these indentations may be difficult to see due to the body's distension with blood.

All hard ticks have a dorsal plate called a shield or scutum, which is absent in soft ticks. In males the scutum is large and covers almost the entire dorsal surface of the body (see Fig. 17.1), whereas in females it is much smaller and is retricted to the anterior part of the body just behind the capitulum (Fig. 17.1). In engorged females the scutum may be difficult to see because it appears small in relation to the enlarged body and becomes pushed forwards so that it is almost vertical in position. The scutum provides a method of immediately recognising hard ticks and also of differentiating between the sexes, although this may not be very important as both sexes bite animals and are therefore potential disease vectors. In the larval and nymphal stages the scutum is small in both sexes.

The body has four pairs of legs terminating in a pair of claws. Although hard ticks are generally dark or light brown, some species have coloured markings on the scutum and body, and sometimes there are shiny patches of colour on the legs; such coloured ticks are referred to as ornate species.

There are no coxal organs in ixodid ticks. Unlike soft ticks, males of some species of hard ticks may have sclerotised plates ventrally, and their number, arrangement and colour may be of taxonomic importance.

Life-cycle

Both the Ixodidae and Argasidae have hemimetabolous life-cycles, that is, there is incomplete metamorphosis involving a larval and nymphal stage. There are, however, important differences between the life-cycles and ecology of ticks in these two families. Adult ixodid ticks remain attached to their hosts for long periods as blood-feeding often lasts for 1–4 weeks. When feeding has finished the enormously engorged tick drops from the host to the ground and seeks shelter under leaves, stones, detritus, amongst surface roots of grasses and shrubs, or buries itself in the surface soil. The time taken for females to digest their blood-meal and commence laying eggs varies according to species and environmental conditions, especially temperature. Sometimes oviposition begins 3–6 days after the female drops from the host, but egg laying may not start until several weeks, or occasionally months, after the end of feeding. Thousands (often 1000–8000) of small spherical eggs are laid in a gelatinous mass which is formed in front and on top of the scutum of the tick (Fig. 17.3). Some species lay as many as 20 000 eggs and the egg mass may become larger than the ovipositing female. Oviposition may last for 10 days, or extend over about 5 weeks. As in argasid ticks the eggs are coated with a waxy secretion produced by Gene's organ, which in the case of ixodid ticks also helps to transfer the eggs

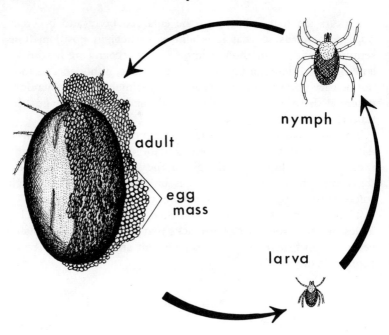

Fig. 17.3 Diagrammatic representation of the life-cycle of an ixodid tick, showing a single nymphal stage, and female with very large mass of eggs.

from the genital opening to the scutum. The ixodid female lays only one batch of eggs, after which she dies.

After about 2–3 weeks to several months six-legged larvae hatch from the eggs. The larvae are minute, being about 0·5–1·5 mm long, and are sometimes referred to as 'seed ticks'. On cursory examination they superficially resemble larval mites, but the presence of a *toothed* hypostome immediately identifies them as ticks. After emergence the larvae remain inactive for a few days after which they swarm over the ground and climb up vegetation and cluster at the tips of grasses and leaves. When suitable hosts pass through a tick-infested habitat the larvae respond to stimuli such as carbon dioxide, host odours, warmth, shadows, vibrations and movements, by waving their front legs in the air. This host-seeking behaviour exhibited by the larvae, and also the nymphs and adults, is called 'questing'. Larvae climb onto their hosts and crawl to their favoured sites for attachment, commonly in the ears or on the eyelids, but the selected site depends on the species of tick and host. The chelicerae and hypostome are inserted deep into the skin of the host and the larvae commence blood-feeding. The larvae remain attached to their hosts for about 3–7 days, and then drop to the ground and seek shelter amongst vegetation or under stones. Larvae normally take 2–7 days to digest their blood-meals, but in cooler weather digestion may extend over several weeks. After all blood has been digested the larvae remain inactive for a few days before they moult to become nymphs.

The newly formed eight-legged nymphs crawl over the ground and climb vegetation and behave similarly to the larvae (that is questing) in seeking out a suitable passing host. They attach themselves to selected sites on the body and begin to feed, and 5–10 days later the fully engorged nymphs drop to the ground and again seek shelter under stones or amongst vegetation. They remain quiescent for about 3–4 weeks, during which time the blood-meal is digested, and afterwards the nymphs moult to produce male or female ixodid tricks. There is only one nymphal stage in the life-cycle of ixodid ticks (Fig. 17.3), whereas argasid ticks have several nymphal stages.

The newly formed adults remain more or less inactive for about 7 days, after which they climb vegetation and start questing for passing hosts. Adult female ixodid ticks take very large blood-meals (e.g. 600 mg of blood), and remain on their hosts for 1–4 weeks. Fully engorged female hard ticks may ingest 200 times their own weight in blood; male ticks take considerably smaller meals. On the ground adult ticks seek shelter under stones, surface vegetation and amongst roots of plants.

Behaviour and habits

Certain species of ixodid tick are more or less host specific. For example, *Boophilus* species feed mainly on cattle, but other species, including many of those of medical importance, are less specific and feed on a wide variety of mammals. Diversity of host species often increases the likelihood of ticks transmitting diseases amongst their hosts, including man. Larvae and nymphs of many, but not all, ticks seem to have a predilection for small animals such as rodents, cats and dogs, and ground-inhabiting birds, whereas adults seem to prefer to feed on cattle, horses and a variety of large and wild mammals. Humans are parasitised by all life-stages of ixodid ticks, but often less so by adults than by the younger stages. The tick's life-cycle may be prolonged by months or even years by lack of suitable hosts. Some species, for example, *Ixodes ricinus*, have a life-cycle which even under favourable conditions lasts about 3 years. In temperate regions development may also be prolonged or cease temporarily during winter months. In warm countries development and breeding may continue throughout the year, but there may be seasonal fluctuations. Adults of some ixodid species may live for up to 7 years.

Although ticks can tolerate considerable variations in temperature and humidity, most species are absent from both very dry and very wet areas, but certain *Hyalomma* species occur in arid areas and deserts. Humidity at soil level can be an important factor in tick survival, and this may be very different from humidities measured at greater heights. Microclimatic conditions at soil level are greatly influenced by the amount and type of ground vegetation; so that the distribution of various species of ticks can often be closely associated with particular types of vegetation.

Both immature and adult ixodid ticks remain on their hosts much longer than do argasid ticks and may be carried many kilometres by their hosts, or even across continents by migrating birds, before they drop off. They are therefore not restricted to their hosts' homes or resting places as are most argasid ticks, but are more widely dispersed.

Three-host ticks

The life-cycle previously described refers to a three-host tick; that is a different individual host, which may be the same or different species, is parasitised by the larva, nymph and adult, and moulting occurs on the ground. Most ixodid ticks have this type of life-cycle, and medically important species of three-host ticks are found in the genera *Ixodes*, *Dermacentor*, *Rhipicephalus* and *Haemaphysalis*. Ticks which feed on three hosts are more likely to become infected with pathogens and be potential vectors of disease than species that feed on one or two hosts.

Two-host ticks

Some species of ticks, in particular many of those in the genera *Hyalomma* and *Rhipicephalus*, are two-host ticks. After the larva has completed feeding it remains on the host and moults to produce a nymph which then feeds on the same host. The engorged nymph drops off, moults and the resultant adult feeds on a different host.

One-host ticks

In a few ticks, such as *Boophilus* species, the larva, nymph and adult all feed on the same host and moulting also takes place on that host. The only stage that leaves the host is the blood-engorged female tick which drops to the ground to lay eggs. One-host ticks are less likely to acquire infections with pathogens than ticks which feed on several hosts, and clearly the only method by which infection can be spread from one host to another by these ticks is by transovarial transmission. One-host ticks are of little or no medical importance, but certain species of *Boophilus* are important vectors of several animal diseases including babesiosis, such as Texas cattle fever (*Babesia bigemina*) and bovine anaplasmosis (*Anaplasma marginale*).

Medical importance

Tick paralysis

Females of certain hard ticks, especially *Dermacentor andersoni* and various species of *Ixodes*, *Hyalomma*, *Rhipicephalus* and *Haemaphysalis*, can cause a condition in man, farm animals, pets and wild animals called tick paralysis. The symptoms appear 5–7 days after a female tick has commenced feeding. There is an acute ascending paralysis affecting the legs with the result that the person cannot walk or stand, and has difficulty in speaking, swallowing and breathing, due to paralysis of the motor nerves. The symptoms are painless and there is very rarely any rise in the patient's temperature. Tick paralysis can be confused with paralysis due to poliomyelitis and certain other paralytic infections. Young children, especially up to the age of 2 years, are most severely affected. Death in animals, and in rare cases also man, can result due to respiratory failure. After ticks have been removed the patient usually makes a full recovery within a few days or weeks.

Tick paralysis is not caused by any pathogens but by various toxins contained in the female tick's saliva which is continually

pumped into the host during the long period the tick is feeding
on the host. Different species of ticks and also different populations of the same species may vary markedly in their ability to
produce tick paralysis in man and animals.

Arboviruses

All arboviruses are transmitted by the tick's bite, and transovarial
transmission commonly occurs.

Russian spring-summer encephalitis (RSSE)
This is caused by one of several closely related viruses of the
RSSE complex which vary in their pathogenicity to man. It is
associated with the taiga forests of Russia, Siberia, northern Asia
and China. The main vector is *Ixodes persulcatus*, but in certain
areas *Haemaphysalis concinna* seems to be an important vector.
After multiplication in the tick, virus accumulates in the salivary
glands, and infection is through the tick's bite. Various small
mammals and birds in addition to ticks serve as reservoirs. There
is a transstadial and transovarial transmission.

Tick-borne (central European) encephalitis (TBE)
This virus produces a disease with symptoms very similar to that
of RSSE. It occurs in central Europe from Scandinavia to the
Balkans. The principal vectors appear to be *Ixodes ricinus* and
Dermacentor marginatus; various small mammals appear to serve
as reservoirs. TBE virus accumulates in the mammary glands of
goats, sheep and cows, and people usually become infected not by
ticks but by drinking infected milk or eating cheese. Both transstadial and transovarial transmission occur.

Omsk haemorrhagic fever (OHF)
This virus produces a disease with symptoms rather similar to
those produced by KFD virus; it occurs in south-western Siberia
and can cause a serious disease, and often death, in muskrat han-
dlers. It was originally thought that ticks were the principal vectors, but it now appears that transmission is mainly by handling
muskrat carcasses, or by eating food contaminated with their
urine or faeces. It seems ticks are not important vectors but
further clarification is needed.

Kyasanur forest disease (KFD)

The disease occurs in tropical forests of southern India and is spread by *Haemaphysalis* species, in particular *H. spinigera*. Small rodents and other mammals including bats and birds may serve as reservoir hosts, while monkeys are likely amplifying hosts. There is transstadial but not apparently transovarial transmission.

Crimean-Congo haemorrhagic fever (CCHF)

Two viruses are included in this group, the most important is Congo virus which occurs in Bulgaria, areas of Russia especially the Crimea, Pakistan and certain areas of West, Central and East Africa. It is transmitted by ticks of the *Hyalomma marginatum* complex, other species of *Hyalomma* and also by *Amblyomma*, *Rhipicephalus* and *Boophilus* species. These ticks occur on a variety of animals, including birds which fly from Russia to Africa, Asia and Western Europe, thus possibly aiding the spread of the disease. Transmission is by tick bite or crushing infected ticks, or by accidental infection when shearing tick-infested sheep. There is transovarial transmission.

Colorado tick fever (CTF)

This is a virus disease which occurs in the USA and Canada and is transmitted to man by *Dermacentor andersoni* and *D. occidentalis*. It is spread amongst rabbits, hares and squirrels, and other rodents, however, by other species of *Dermacentor*, and also by *Haemaphysalis* and the argasid tick *Otobius lagophilus*. Both rodents and ticks form the reservoirs of the virus. Transovarial transmission probably occurs.

Miscellaneous arboviruses

Ixodid ticks spread many other arboviruses to man, including Powassan encephalitis (POW) virus in North America, Langat (LGT) virus in Malaysia, Kemerovo fever (KEM) virus in Siberia, and Quaranfil fever (QRF) in Egypt. Louping ill (LI), an important virus disease of sheep in Britain, is spread by *Ixodes ricinus*, and is occasionally acquired by humans.

Rickettsiae

Rocky Mountain spotted fever (RMSF)

This disease is also known as Mexican spotted fever, Sâo Paulo spotted fever, American tick-borne typhus and by several other local names. Different strains of the causative organism, *Rickettsia rickettsii*, vary considerably in their virulence. Rocky Mountain spotted fever occurs in North, Central and South America, where it can cause death in man. The principal vectors in North America are *Dermacentor andersoni* and *D. variabilis*. Dogs, rabbits and small rodents also become infected and the disease is spread amongst them by various species of ticks belonging to several genera. Various animals may act as reservoirs of the disease, but as they remain infectious for relatively short periods, the main reservoir is the tick, in which the rickettsiae can survive during the winter. In South America *Amblyomma* species are the main vectors.

There is an incubation period of about 9–12 days before an infected tick becomes infective, and transmission is normally through the bite of any stage in the life-cycle of the tick. An infective tick, however, must remain feeding on a host for at least 2 hours before sufficient rickettsiae are injected into the host for the host to become infected. Consequently, early tick removal may prevent transmission. More rarely transmission is through tick faeces, or by crushing ticks in the fingers and accidentally rubbing the rickettsiae into the eyes or abrasions. There is transvarial and transstadial transmission.

Siberian tick typhus (STT)

This disease is similar to Rocky Mountain spotted fever, and the causative organism, *Rickettsia sibirica*, is antigenically close to *R. rickettsii*. It occurs in Russia, Pacific areas and on the Japanese islands. Vectors include species of *Dermacentor*, *Haemaphysalis*, *Rhipicephalus* and *Hyalomma*. Infection is by tick bites, and both transstadial and transovarial transmission occur. Ticks appear to be the main reservoir of infection. Mammals, mainly rodents, may also serve as reservoirs, but since infection in these animals is short-lived they are probably not important in maintaining the reservoir. Birds may also be minor reservoirs.

Boutonneuse fever

Also known as fièvre boutonneuse, Marseilles fever, South African tick typhus, Kenyan tick typhus, Indian tick typhus, Crimean tick typhus, etc., this disease is caused by *Rickettsia conori*. The symptoms in man are similar to those caused by Rocky Mountain spotted fever. It occurs in the Mediterranean region, the Middle East, Crimea, most of India, Southern Asia and Africa. One of the principal vectors is *Rhipicephalus sanguineus*, the dog tick, but it appears that ticks of most ixodid genera can transmit the disease to man. Transmission is by the tick's bite, and both transstadial and transovarial transmission occur. Infection can also occur if infected ticks are crushed and the rickettsiae rubbed into abrasions or in the eyes. Both ticks and rodent serve as reservoirs, the role of dogs as a reservoir needs clarification.

Miscellaneous rickettsiae

A disease known as Queensland tick typhus (*R. australis*) is transmitted by *Ixodes* ticks and occurs in the Queensland area of Australia.

Another rickettsial disease is Q-fever (*Coxiella burneti*) which has a world-wide distribution and is mainly a disease of rodents and other mammals. It is mainly spread by consuming contaminated milk and meat from cattle, and the inhalation of dried infected faeces by those working with cattle. Hard ticks may help maintain an enzootic cycle, and possibly even transmit the disease to man. Transovarial transmission occurs.

A few other non-pathogenic or apparently unimportant rickettsiae have been isolated from ticks. In addition to causing human diseases, ixodid ticks are also vectors of several rickettsiae of veterinary importance to animals such as cattle, sheep and dogs.

Spirochaetes

Lyme disease, which was first recognised in 1975 in the USA, is caused by a spirochaete transmitted in the eastern USA by *Ixodes dammini*, whose more normal hosts are deer, and by *I. pacificus* in western USA. Symptoms include arthritic pains in the joints. Little is known about the epidemiology of this non-fatal disease, but in addition to the USA it has appeared in Canada, Europe, Russia and Australia. There is both transovarial and transstadial transmission.

Tularaemia

A bacterial disease caused by *Pasteurella tularensis* which occurs in North America, Europe, Japan and Asia and infects mainly rabbits, but other rodents and even birds can be infected. The disease is spread by a variety of direct contact methods such as handling infected live animals, carcasses, drinking contaminated water, eating raw or uncooked meats and also by the bite of various hard ticks. *Chrysops discalis* is also a vector (see p. 123).

Control

Methods for the removal of argasid ticks described on p. 222 are also applicable to the removal of ixodid ticks, which if not removed may remain attached for several days or even weeks. The types of insect repellents described on p. 222 can also be used to prevent attachment of ixodid ticks.

Various insecticidal formulations can be applied to domestic pets, such as dogs, to rid them of their ticks. Recommended treatments include solutions of 0·5 per cent malathion, 0·1 per cent dichlorvos (DDVP), 1 per cent carbaryl (Sevin), 0·1 per cent dioxathion, 0·2 per cent naled (Dibrom) and 1·0 per cent coumaphos. Alternatively, dusts of 5 per cent carbaryl or 0·5 per cent coumaphos, 3–5 per cent malathion or 1 per cent trichlorphon can be applied to the coats of pets. Floors of houses, porches, verandahs and other sites where infected pets sleep should be sprayed with oil solutions or emulsions of organochlorine or organophosphate insecticides, such as 1 per cent propoxur (Baygon), 0·5 per cent diazinon, 2 per cent malathion, 5 per cent carbaryl (Sevin), or 0·5 per cent chlorpyrifos (Dursban). This will kill ticks still attached to hosts as well as those that have dropped off. Ultra-low-volume (ULV) spraying with propoxur at the rate of about $0·5–2·0 \, \text{kg/ha}^{-1}$ may give good tick control for about 6 weeks.

The dipping of sheep and cattle, and sometimes other domestic livestock, in acaricidal baths, or spraying them with insecticides, is often crucial if ticks and tick-borne diseases of man as well as of livestock are to be effectively controlled.

Intensive use of insecticides to control veterinary important ticks has resulted in ticks in many parts of the world becoming resistant to a wide range of insecticides—organochlorines, organophosphates, carbamates and even sometimes synthetic pyrethroids.

Chapter 18
Scabies Mites

The scabies or itch mite which occurs on man belongs to the species *Sarcoptes scabiei* and has a world-wide distribution. Similar mites which cannot be reliably separated from *S. scabiei* are found on numerous wild and domesticated animals but such mites very rarely infect man. They are probably the same species as occurs on man but are physiologically adapted to life on non-human hosts.

Scabies mites are not vectors of any disease but cause the conditions known in man as scabies, acariasis, Norwegian itch, crusted scabies or seven-year itch.

External morphology

The female mite is just about visible without the aid of a hand lens (0·30–0·45 mm). It is whitish and disc-shaped. Dorsally the mite is covered with numerous small peg-like protuberances and a few bristles, and both dorsally and ventrally there are series of

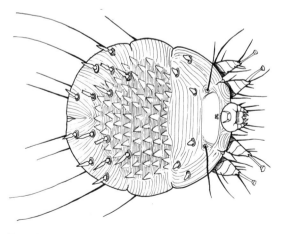

Fig. 18.1 Dorsal view of an adult mature female scabies mite, *Sarcoptes scabiei*.

lines across the body giving the mite a striated appearance (Fig. 18.1). Adults have four pairs of short and cylindrical legs divided into five apparent ring-like segments. The first two pairs of legs end in short stalks called pedicels which terminate in thin-walled roundish structures often termed 'suckers'. In the females the posterior two pairs of legs do not have 'suckers' but end in long and very conspicuous bristles.

There is no real distinct head, but the short and fat palps and pincer-like chelicerae of the mouthparts protrude anteriorly from the body.

Adult male scabies mites are only about 0·20–0·25 mm long, and apart from their small size may also be distinguished from females by the presence of 'suckers' on the last pairs of legs (Fig. 18.2).

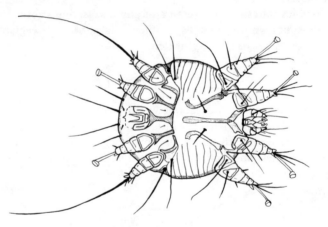

Fig. 18.2 Ventral view of an adult male *Sarcoptes scabiei* showing 'suckers' on last pair of legs.

Life-cycle

The female scabies mite selects places on the body where the skin is thin and wrinkled, such as between the fingers, wrists, elbows, feet, penis, scrotum, buttocks and axillae. The majority (63 per cent) of mites are found on the hands and wrists and about 11 per cent occur on the elbows. The mite digs and eats her way into the surface layers of the skin—the stratum corneum. In women mites may often be found burrowing beneath and around the breasts and nipples. In young children whose skin is soft and tender they may be found burrowing on the face and other parts of the body, and often the greatest number of mites on children up to a year old are found on the feet. When the females have burrowed into the superficial layers of the skin they excavate winding tunnels at the rate of about 1–5 mm per day, which are seen on the skin as very thin twisting lines a few millimetres to several centimetres long. The mite feeds on liquids oozing from dermal cells she has chewed. She lays 1–3 eggs a day in her tunnel.

The eggs hatch within 3–5 days and small six-legged larvae emerge which look like miniature adults. These larvae crawl out of the tunnels onto the surface of the skin where a large number die, but a few succeed in either burrowing into the stratum corneum or entering a hair follicle to produce not a tunnel but a small pocket called a 'moulting pocket'. After 2–3 days the larva moults in the pocket to produce an eight-legged nymph. A nymph destined to become a female mite moults to produce a sexually immature female which remains more or less quiescent in the moulting pocket until she is fertilised by a male, after which she enlarges in size to become a mature (ovigerous) female. Mating may be accomplished by the male either burrowing through the surface of the skin into the moulting pocket containing the female, or on the surface of the skin. Only after fertilisation does the female commence to burrow through the skin, and after about 3–5 days she starts to lay eggs in the tunnel. Female mites very rarely leave their burrows.

The life-cycle from egg to adult takes about 11–20 days. Female scabies mites may live about 1–2 months on man, away from man they may survive for about 7–10 days under ideal conditions, but they usually live only 2–4 days.

In the life-cycle of the male mite the six-legged larva moults to become a nymph which stays in the moulting pocket until it changes into an adult male, this stage being reached 4–6 days after the eggs have hatched. Adult males, which are about half the size of mature female mites, can be found in either very short burrows (usually less than 1 mm) or in small pockets in the skin. However, they probably spend most of their life wandering around on the surface of the skin seeking females awaiting to be fertilised.

Scabies is a contagious complaint which is transmitted only by close contact. It is therefore a family disease spreading amongst those living in close association, especially when they sleep together in the same bed. It can be spread amongst courting couples who are habitually holding hands. It appears that the actual transfer of mites from person to person takes about 15–20 minutes of close contact. The incidence of scabies often increases during wars and disasters, such as earthquakes, floods and famines when people are sleeping and living in very overcrowded situations. It is also possible to get infected by sleeping in a bed formerly occupied by an infected person, but experimental work has indicated that this rarely happens. It is therefore not usually worthwhile fumigating or sterilising clothing or bedclothes to prevent scabies spreading, but in epidemics, or in cases of Norwegian or crusted scabies resulting from the use of immunosuppressive drugs, such measures may be needed. Ten minutes at 50°C will kill the mites, alternatively clothing and bedding can be kept unused for about 4 days, which usually results in their death. Laundering will also kill any mites on clothing.

Recognition of scabies

Scabies in man can be diagnosed by detection of the female mite's thin twisting tunnels, which are easier to see on fair-skinned than on dark-skinned people. The faeces deposited in the tunnels may be visible through the skin and appear as pepper-like spots. However, for those with less experience in scabies detection, a more reliable procedure is to remove and identify the mites. The surface layers of the skin at the end of the tunnels should be gently scratched away with sharp dissecting needles and the mites, which usually readily adhere to the points of the needles, removed and examined under a × 50 magnification.

The average number of mature adult female scabies mites found on a person is about 11; most patients have 1–15 mites, only about 3 per cent have more than 50 mites.

The scabies rash

This is a follicular papular eruption that occurs mainly on areas of the body not infected with burrowing mites, such as the buttocks and around the waist and the shoulders, but the rash can also occur on other parts of the body such as the arms, calves and ankles. It does not appear on the head, centre of the chest or back, nor on the palms of the hands or soles of the feet. The rash is produced in response to the patient being sensitised, that is the rash is an allergic reaction produced by the mites. Frequently a patient is unaware he is harbouring mites until a rash appears.

When a person is infected for the first time with itch mites the rash does not appear until about 4–6 weeks later, but in individuals who have previously been infected a rash may develop within a few days after reinfection. The rash may persist for several weeks after all scabies mites have been destroyed. The severe pruritus which soon develops results in vigorous and constant scratching, especially at night, and this frequently leads to the development of secondary bacterial infections. These may be quite severe leading to boils, pustules, ecthyma, eczema and impetigo contagiosa. These complications tend to mask the nature of the complaint, and as a consequence correct diagnosis of scabies may not be made. The seriousness of the symptoms is not always directly related to the number of mites, and severe reactions may be found on people harbouring few mites.

The condition in Europe known as Norwegian or crusted scabies is rare but highly contagious due to the vast numbers of mites in the exfoliating scales. It is characterised by the formation of thick keralatic crusts over the hands and feet, scaling eruptions on other parts of the body, and usually large numbers of mites, but a much less pronounced degree of itching. It is not clear why the condition develops, but it may be due to a loss of immunity in man which allows the establishment of enormous numbers of mites. This hypothesis is supported by the finding that the development of Norwegian scabies has sometimes been associated with the extensive use of corticosteroids. This reduces irritation and consequently reduces the patient's scratching, an act which helps in the removal and destruction of some mites.

Treatment of scabies

All cases of scabies can be cured, there are no resistant infections. Methods aimed at killing the mites will do little to immediately alleviate the nuisance and irritation caused by the rash, although this will eventually disappear. Separate medical treatment, however, may be necessary especially if secondary infections have become established. In the past, a common procedure was to give the patient a hot bath and vigorous scrubbing with a brush until he bled, but this is not very effective at either removing or killing the mites. However, as many, but certainly not all, patients with scabies are dirty, an ordinary bath before treatment may be advisable for general hygienic reasons. However, if large numbers of patients suffering from scabies are to be treated, such as in epidemic situations, bathing may not be practical.

A 20–25 per cent benzyl benzoate emulsion can be painted on a patient from the neck downwards, and after allowing some 5–10 minutes for this application to dry the patient can re-dress. A single efficient treatment should in most cases result in a complete eradication of the mites, but a repeat treatment on the third day may be advisable. Only in rare cases does dermatitis result from the use of benzyl benzoate and this is more likely to happen in young children.

Mitigal is a yellowish oily liquid sulphur preparation which is painted undiluted over the body from the neck downwards. A single treatment should be 100 per cent effective. A mild form of dermatitis may be produced in some people. Tetmosol is another sulphur compound sometimes used to treat scabies. It is slow in its action and usually about three treatments 24 hours apart are recommended for a complete cure. It is therefore of limited use in mass treatments. It has been combined with soap and sold as Tetmosol soap, and in this form, when regularly used in washing and bathing, it has a slow curative effect and also acts as a prophylactic.

Although these two sulphur preparations and benzyl benzoate are still used, a better treatment for scabies consists of applying a 1 per cent HCH cream or lotion to the body, but this is not always available in sufficient quantities to treat large numbers of people. Although, as with benzyl benzoate and Mitigal, a single treatment has a high success rate, a second application 2–7 days later, if this is possible, ensures a complete cure. More recently 1 per cent malathion has been used, and as with HCH a single treatment is usually sufficient. Crotamiton applied as a 10 per cent cream or lotion is a very safe treatment, but 2–5 daily applications are needed.

With a highly contagious condition like scabies it is important to treat all members of a family or community living in close association, not just the individual with a particularly bad infestation of mites, otherwise reinfestation will soon occur.

Chapter 19
Scrub Typhus Mites

There are more than 1200 species of trombiculid mites belonging to several genera but only a few species attack man. Larvae of trombiculid mites are often called red bugs or chiggers. The Trombiculidae have a more or less world-wide distribution in temperate and tropical regions, but the medically important species, such as the *Leptrombidium deliense* group, *L. akamushi* and *L. fletcheri*, are found only in Asia. Certain species are vectors of scrub typhus (*Rickettsia tsutsugamushi*) in parts of Asiatic Russia, India, Sri Lanka to South-east Asia, Burma, China, Korea, Japan, Taiwan, New Guinea and northern Australia, etc.

Other trombiculid mites in many parts of the world cause itching and a form of dermatitis in man, known as scrub-itch or trombidiosis. In Europe larvae of *Neotrombicula autumnalis*, although not disease vectors, often attack man and are frequently known as harvest mites.

External morphology

Adults and nymphs

Adults are small mites (1·0–2·0 mm), usually reddish and covered dorsally and ventrally with numerous feathered hairs giving them a velvety appearance. There are four pairs of legs ending in paired claws. The body is distinctly constricted between the third and fourth pairs of legs giving it an outline resembling a figure of eight. The palps and mouthparts project in front of the body and are clearly visible from above (Fig. 19.1).

The nymph resembles the adult but is smaller (0·5–1·0 mm) and the body is less densely covered with feathered hairs.

Neither the adults nor nymphs are of direct medical importance; they do not bite man or animals but feed on small arthropods and their eggs. It is only the larvae which are parasitic and hence responsible for the spread of diseases.

241

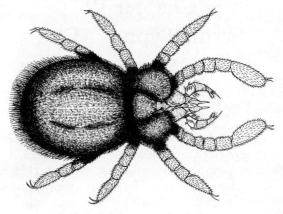

Fig. 19.1 Dorsal view of an adult trombiculid mite of the genus *Leptotrombidium*.

Larvae

Larvae are very small (0·15–0·3 mm), but after engorging they may increase sixfold in size, they are usually reddish or orange but may be pale yellow or straw-coloured. There are three pairs of legs which terminate in a pair of relatively large claws. Both legs and body are covered with fine featured hairs. The five-segmented palps and mouthparts are large and conspicuous, giving

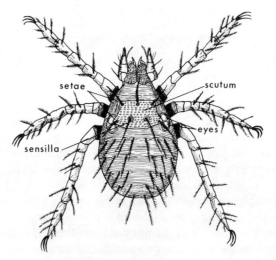

Fig. 19.2 Dorsal view of a larval trombiculid mite of the genus *Leptotrombidium*. Note scutum, paired sensillae and five scutal setae.

the larvae the appearance of having a false head (Fig. 19.2). Dorsally and on the anterior part of the body there is a rectangular or pentagonal-shaped scutum bearing three to six setae. However, as the scutum is weakly sclerotised it is often difficult to see under the microscope, unless the light is correctly aligned. More easily detected are a pair of eyes on either side of the scutum. In medically important species there are five feathered setae on the scutum and in addition a pair of specialised feathered hairs known as sensillae which arise from distinct bases. The combination of a body covered with feathered hairs, five scutal hairs, a pair of flagelliform sensillae and large pigmented eyes distinguishes larvae of *Leptotrombium* from larvae of other mite genera.

Life-cycle

Adult trombiculid mites are not parasitic but live in the soil feeding on a variety of small soil-inhabiting arthropods and their eggs. A female mite lays one to five spherical eggs each day on the surface of damp soil or under leaves. In hot climates egg laying continues uninterrupted for a year or more, but in cooler areas of South-east Asia, including Japan, oviposition apparently ceases during the cooler months of the year, and adults enter into partial or complete hibernation.

After about 5–7 days the egg shell splits, although the six-legged larva does not emerge but remains within the egg shell and is called the deutovum. After about 5–7 days the larva crawls out of the egg shell and usually becomes very active and swarms over the ground and climbs up grasses and other low-lying vegetation. Larvae attach themselves to birds or mammals, including man, walking through infested vegetation. When the larval mites have climbed onto a suitable host they congregate where the skin is soft and moist, such as the ears, genitalia and around the anus. On man larvae seek out areas where clothing is tight against the skin, such as around the waist or the ankles.

Larvae pierce the host's skin with their powerful mouthparts and inject saliva into the wound which causes disintegration of the cells. Larvae do not normally suck up blood, rather lymph and other fluid and semi-digested materials. The repeated injection of saliva into the wound produces a skin reaction in the host and the formation of a peculiar tube-like structure which extends vertically downwards in the host's skin, and is known as the stylostome or hypostome. Some trombiculid mites remain attached to their hosts for as long as 1 month, but the *Leptotrombidium* vectors of scrub typhus remain on man for only about 2–10 days. The engorged larva drops to the ground and buries itself just below the surface of the soil or underneath debris.

The larva having concealed itself becomes quiescent and this stage is known as the protonymph. After 7–10 days the protonymph moults to produce an eight-legged reddish nymph covered with feathered hairs. The nymphs are not parasitic, but feed on soil-inhabiting arthropods. After a period of some days to about 2 weeks the nymph ceases feeding and becomes inactive, and is called a preadult, which after about another 14 days moults to give rise to an adult. The adults resemble the nymphs but are larger, and like them are free-living and feed on small soil animals.

The life-cycle usually takes about 2–3 months but may be as long as 8–10 months. The stages in the life-cycle can be summarised as follows (the inactive stages are bracketed): egg→(deutovum)→larva→(protonymph)→nymph→(preadult)→adult.

Ecology

The free-living nymphs and adults of *Leptotrombidium* have specialised ecological requirements. For example, habitats must contain sufficient numbers of suitable arthropod fauna to serve as food. The habitat must also be one in which host animals such as rodents regularly traverse so that larvae will have opportunities of attaching themselves to their hosts. Wild rats of the genus *Rattus*, subgenus *Rattus*, are very important hosts of *Leptotrombidium* larvae. In Japan, and possibly elsewhere, small rodents such as species of *Apodemus* and *Microtus* and other subgenera of *Rattus* are also important hosts. Domestic rats play little or no part in the ecology or epidemiology of scrub typhus. In addition to hosts such as these, which maintain the mite population in an area, other more or less incidental hosts may be important in aiding the dispersal of larvae to other areas.

Relatively small changes in moisture content of the soil, temperature and humidity can be crucial, as they may cause adults to bury deeper into the soil and cease egg laying. Habitats favouring the survival and development of the nymphs and adults are therefore in a very delicate ecological balance. Frequently only very small areas of ground, often just a few square metres, prove to be suitable habitats. This can result in a very patchy distribution of *Leptotrombidium* mites over small areas, but in some situations habitats may comprise several square kilometres. Areas suitable for mite survival and development are often called 'mite islands', a term which emphasises their frequent isolation from other ecologically suitable areas.

Medical importance

Nuisance

Several species of Trombiculidae attack man in temperate and tropical regions of the world. Although such mites are not responsible for transmitting any disease, they can nevertheless cause intense itching and irritation, commonly referred to as 'harvest-bug itch', 'autumnal itch' or 'scrub itch'. Larval mites commonly attack the legs. If they are forcibly removed, their mouthparts frequently remain imbedded in the skin and this may promote further irritation. People usually become infested with these mites after walking through long grass or scrub vegetation.

Scrub typhus

The causative organism is *Rickettsia tsutsugamushi* and the disease is commonly known as scrub typhus, mite-borne typhus, rural typhus, Japanese river fever or tsutsugamushi disease. The disease is restricted to Asia and occurs over a large area, extending from the Primorye regions of Russia, India, Sri Lanka, Burma, Korea, Malaysia, South-East Asia, China, Taiwan, Japan, Philippines and New Guinea to northern Australia and the neighbouring South-west Pacific islands south to about the tropic of Capricorn. Although most cases are reported from low-lying areas, infections occur up to a height of 1000 m in many areas, and even up to about 2000 m in Taiwan and 3200 m in the Himalayas. In India, *Leptotrombidium* mites have been found at elevations of 2700 m. During the Second World War (1939–45) the incidence of scrub typhus in troops in the Asiatic–Pacific areas was second only to malaria.

Scrub typhus has often been regarded as a zoonosis, but

although *R. tsutsugamushi* occurs in forest and rural rodents and *Tupaia* (tree-shrews), it appears that these animals have a minor role, if any, in the maintenance of scrub typhus. Experimentally it has been shown that it is often difficult to infect trombiculid larvae by feeding them on infected rodents, and even if they do become infected the rickettsiae may not be transovarially transmitted to their progeny. It appears that larvae infected by feeding on man can pass the infection to their own progeny by transovarial transmission, and subsequently to man and rodents. *Leptotrombidium* mites themselves are the main reservoirs of infection.

Man becomes infected following the bite of infected larval trombiculid mites, especially *Leptotrombidium akamushi* and the *L. deliense* group of species. People usually get bitten when they visit or work in areas having so-called mite islands, that is patches of vegetation harbouring large numbers of host-seeking larvae. These mite islands may be at the edge of the forest or bush, or on cleared and cultivated land which harbours rodents and is also suitable for the survival and development of the mites. The disease is often associated with 'fringe habitats', that is habitats separating two major vegetation zones such as forests and plantations, because these areas are often heavily populated with rodent hosts. The risk of scrub typhus transmission is often related to the number of areas of different types of vegetation, that is habitat diversity.

All known foci of scrub typhus are characterised by natural or man-made changes in environmental conditions. The very close association between: (a) *Leptotrombidium* mites, (b) wild rodents such as *Rattus* (*Rattus*), (c) transitional secondary vegetation, for example, grass, shrubs and saplings, and (d) *R. tsutsugamushi* has been described as a 'zoonotic tetrad of chigger-borne rickettsiosis'.

Because larval mites attach themselves to only a single host during their life-cycle the disease cannot be spread by larvae feeding on an infected host (e.g. man) then another. The infection acquired by mites feeding on hosts with rickettsiae is passed on to the free-living nymphal stages and then to the free-living adults. When the female lays her eggs they are infected with rickettsiae and this infection is passed on to the emerging larvae. So, although they have not previously fed on man they are already infected and consequently transmit the disease to their hosts (man or rodents) when they feed for the first and only time. This inherited type of transmission is called transovarial transmission and can be maintained for several mite generations before the rickettsiae are reduced in numbers and finally disappear.

Control

The application to the body of suitable insect repellents such as dimethyl phthalate, diethyltoluamide, dibutyl phthalate, ethyl hexanediol and benzyl benzoate may be of help in reducing the likelihood of people getting infected with mites. Clothing can also be impregnated with suitable repellents.

If mite islands can be identified then it may be possible to remove the scrub vegetation mechanically or by herbicides, and so ensure that the habitat is no longer suitable for the survival of the mites. This, however, frequently is not possible, especially if mites are inhabiting cultivated land where ground vegetation consists mainly of crops. Spraying areas known or suspected of harbouring mites with residual insecticides such as DDT, HCH, dieldrin, fenthion (Baytex), malathion, propoxur (Baygon), toxaphene (camphechlor), diazinon or other insecticides, preferably as fogs or emulsions, can do much to reduce the mite population. Insecticidal sprays can be applied from knapsack sprayers, or from equipment mounted on vehicles or aircraft which generates insecticidal aerosols or fogs. Ultra-low-volume spraying has also been used in some areas.

Chapter 20
Miscellaneous Mites

Demodex folliculorum

It was originally believed that there was just a single species of *Demodex* associated with man, namely *Demodex folliculorum*, but it is now known there are two species. *Demodex folliculorum* (Fig. 20.1) is the more elongate species (0·2–0·4 mm) and inhabits the hair follicles, while *D. brevis* is a squatter species (0·1–0·2 mm) living in the sebaceous glands. Both species have a striated body and four pairs of very short stubby legs and are remarkably non-mite like.

Demodex mites are therefore found in hair follicles or sebaceous glands, where they feed on subcutaneous tissues, especially sebum. They are particularly common on the nose, eyelids and cheeks adjacent to the nose. They have also been found in ear wax and in the extruded contents of comedones ('blackheads'). Females lay eggs within the hair follicles and these hatch to produce six-legged larvae which moult to give rise to nymphs and finally adults. All the developmental stages, which extend over 13–15 days, occur within the hair follicles or sebaceous glands. Little is known about their biology but apparently a high proportion of adults, especially women, unknowingly have these mites. They are rarely found on children or adolescents.

Normally they do not appear to produce any adverse effects, although possibly they may sometimes cause dermatitis, such as acne, rosacea, impetigo contagiosa or blepharites. Daily washing

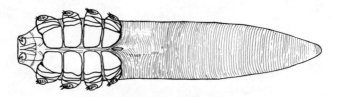

Fig. 20.1 Dorsal view of *Demodex folliculorum*, the hair follicle mite, showing four small stumpy legs.

with soap and water can reduce infections. In severe infections resulting in dermatitis 'Danish ointment', which contains a compound polysulphide, can be used, but this should not be applied to the eyelids otherwise irritation may occur. Alternative treatments consist of applying 0·5 per cent selenium sulphide cream, 10 per cent sulphur, or 0·5 per cent HCH cream ('Kwell').

Dermatophagoides pteronyssinus

This mite has a more or less world-wide distribution. It is very small (0·3 mm) and is generally known as the house-dust mite (Fig. 20.2). It lives amongst bed clothes, mattresses, carpets and general house dust. The life-cycle, egg to adult, takes about 3 weeks. They are very rarely seen although the allergic symptoms they, and their faeces, produce such as asthma and rhinitis may

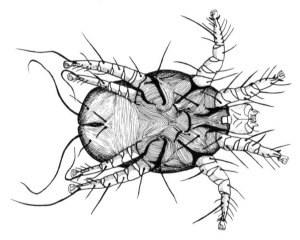

Fig. 20.2 Ventral view of one of the house dust mites, *Dermatophagoides pteronyssinus*.

be quite common. They feed on discarded skin scales, scurf and other organic debris. A survey in Holland showed that all houses examined harboured these mites. Typically there may be 11–30 mites/g^{-1} of house dust, but as many as 3500 mites/g^{-1} have been recorded. After bed-making there may be 0·04–0·34 mites/m^{-3} of air.

Other mites

There are numerous other mites which are parasitic on mammals and birds, including pets and livestock, and some of them occasionally become parasitic on man. For example, the cosmopolitan tropical rat mite (*Ornithonyssus bacoti*), the tropical fowl mite (*O. bursa*), and the chicken mite (*Dermanyssus gallinae*) may sometimes infect people, especially those working closely with infected animals. Their bites can cause irritation and dermatitis.

There are also other mites that live amongst stored products, grains and animal feeds, and people habitually handling these substances may develop allergic symptoms such as dermatitis, and more rarely bronchitis and asthma. This may lead to terms such as 'grocer's itch', 'straw or hay itch' and 'copra itch' to describe these occupational hazards.

Further Reading

ALEXANDER J. O'D. (1984) *Arthropods and Human Skin.* Springer-Verlag, Berlin.

BUSVINE J. R. (1980) *Insects and Hygiene. The Biology and Control of Insect Pests of Medical and Domestic Importance.* Chapman and Hall, London.

HARWOOD R. F. & JAMES M. T. (1979) *Entomology in Human and Animal Health.* Macmillan, New York.

KETTLE D. S. (1984) *Medical and Veterinary Entomology.* Croom Helm, London.

MARSHALL A. G. (1981) *The Ecology of Ectoparasitic Insects.* Academic Press, London.

MELLANBY K. (1972) *Scabies.* E. W. Classey, Middlesex.

NASH T. A. M. (1969) *Africa's Bane. The Tsetse Fly.* Collins, London.

ORKIN M. & MAIBACH H. I. eds. (1985) *Cutaneous Infestations and Insect Bites.* Dermatology series **No. 4,** Marcel Dekker, New York.

SERVICE M. W. (1980) *A Guide to Medical Entomology.* Macmillan, London.

SERVICE M. W. (1986) *Blood-sucking Insects. Vectors of Disease.* (Studies in Biology Series, No. 167) Edward Arnold, London.

SMITH K. V. G., ed. (1973) *Insects and other Arthropods of Medical Importance.* British Musem (Natural History), London.

WARE G. W. (1983) *Pesticides. Theory and Application.* W. H. Freeman & Co., San Francisco.

WORLD HEALTH ORGANIZATION (1980) Resistance of vectors of disease to pesticides. *World Health Organization Technical Report Series,* **No. 655.**

WORLD HEALTH ORGANIZATION (1982) Biological control of vectors of disease. *World Health Organization Technical Report Series,* **No. 679.**

WORLD HEALTH ORGANIZATION (1983) Integrated vector control. *World Health Organization Technical Report Series,* **No. 688.**

WORLD HEALTH ORGANIZATION (1984) Chemical methods for the control of arthropod vectors and pests of public health importance. *World Health Organization, Geneva.*

WORLD HEALTH ORGANIZATION (1985) Arthropod-borne and rodent-borne viral diseases. *World Health Organization Technical Report Series,* **No. 719.**

YOUDEOWEI A. & SERVICE M. W. (1983) *Pest and Vector Management in the Tropics.* Longman, London.

Index